Infertility
and the Novels
of Sophie Cottin

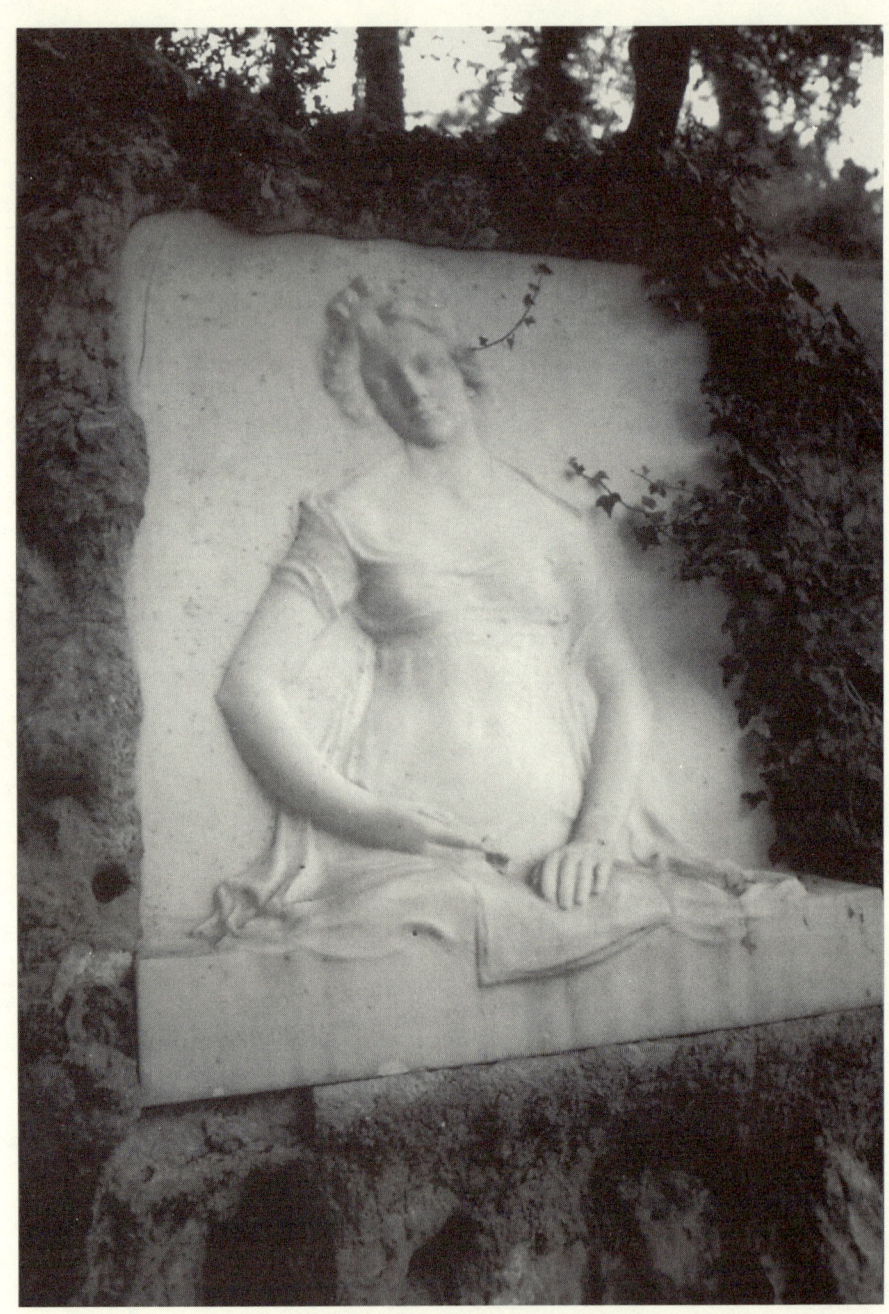

Monument to Sophie Cottin, Jean Escoula, 1910, Allées Fernand de Cardailhac, Bagnères-de-Bigorre, France. Photograph Michael J. Call.

Infertility and the Novels of Sophie Cottin

Michael J. Call

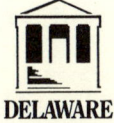

Newark: University of Delaware Press
London: Associated University Presses

© 2002 by Rosemont Publishing & Printing Corp.

All rights reserved. Authorization to photocopy items for internal or personal use, or the internal or personal use of specific clients, is granted by the copyright owner, provided that a base fee of $10.00, plus eight cents per page, per copy is paid directly to the Copyright Clearance Center, 222 Rosewood Drive, Danvers, Massachusetts 01923. [0-87413-807-8/02 $10.00 + 8¢ pp, pc.]

Other than as indicated in the foregoing, this book may not be reproduced, in whole or in part, in any form (except as permitted by Sections 107 and 108 of the U.S. Copyright Law, and except for brief quotes appearing in reviews in the public press).

Associated University Presses
2010 Eastpark Boulevard
Cranbury, NJ 08512

Associated University Presses
16 Barter Street
London WC1A 2AH, England

Associated University Presses
P.O. Box 338, Port Credit
Mississauga, Ontario
Canada L5G 4L8

The paper used in this publication meets the requirements of the American National Standard for Permanence of Paper for Printed Library Materials Z39.48-1984.

Library of Congress Cataloging-in-Publication Data

Call, Michael J.
    Infertility and the novels of Sophie Cottin / Michael J. Call.
      p. cm.
    Includes bibliographical references and index.
    ISBN 0-87413-807-8 (alk. paper)
      1. Cottin, Madame (Sophie), 1770–1807—Criticism and interpretation.
    2. Infertility, Female, in literature. I. Title.
PQ2211.C412 Z56   2002
843'.6—dc21   2002072462

PRINTED IN THE UNITED STATES OF AMERICA

To Connie

Contents

Acknowledgments	9
Introduction	13
1. The Early Life of Sophie Cottin	17
2. Infertility and Plenitude in *Claire d'Albe*	50
3. Back in Step with Jean-Jacques: *Malvina*	71
4. The Anger of *Amélie Mansfield*	82
5. *Mathilde* and the Miracle of Bagnères	102
6. Filial Devotion in *Elisabeth*	135
Conclusion	153
Notes	158
Bibliography	163
Index	166

Acknowledgments

I WISH TO ACKNOWLEDGE THE HELP AND ENCOURAGEMENT I HAVE received from several sources in the completion of this project. Brigham Young University's Women's Research Institute was especially helpful in the initial phase, funding a trip to the Bibliothèque Nationale in Paris to begin my research. I am also grateful for a travel to collections grant awarded by the National Endowment for the Humanities.

The College of Humanities at BYU has been generous in giving me time off from teaching duties to complete the manuscript as well as funding a trip to Bagnères-de-Bigorre, the town at the foot of the Pyrenees that was, as the reader will see, a site of great significance in Sophie Cottin's life.

Erica Harth of Brandeis University, director of an NEH summer seminar I participated in at Radcliffe College, Boston, was especially helpful in reviewing early versions of my analysis of Cottin's first novel, *Claire d'Albe*. I also thank the editors of *Eighteenth-Century Fiction* for their encouragement and the permission to include here much of the material on *Claire d'Albe* that first appeared in the January 1995 volume of their journal.

Several individuals have assisted along the way with research and editing—in particular, Daryl P. Lee, Lauri Westerberg Haddock, Michelle Dixon-McDonald, Rebecca Isom Call, Michael Josiah Call, and Corey B. Chipman.

Special thanks go to Vincent and Denise Merle d'Aubigné—direct descendants of Jeanne Cottin, Sophie's sister-in-law—who, upon learning I was writing a book on Sophie, graciously invited my wife and me to their home in Fontainebleau where we spent a marvelous afternoon sharing family stories. The Merle d'Aubignés truly represent all that is best in France.

I am most of all indebted to my wife Connie, whose experience with infertility helped me understand Sophie Cottin better when I met her.

Infertility
and the Novels
of Sophie Cottin

Introduction

Thus, towards the end of the eighteenth century a change came about which, if I were rewriting history, I should describe more fully and think of greater importance than the Crusades or the Wars of the Roses. The middle-class woman began to write.
—Virginia Woolf, *A Room of One's Own*

Sophie Cottin's story, little known to modern readers on either side of the Atlantic, may nevertheless be a perfect case study of a woman's "coming to writing" in postrevolutionary France. Like many French women novelists of her time, she was appreciated by a wide and diverse reading audience, enjoying a popularity that endured long after her death in 1807. Even Sainte-Beuve, no fan of women writers, grudgingly acknowledged: "Rien n'égale le succès qu'eurent dans leur temps les romans de madame Cottin" ["Nothing equals the success Madame Cottin's novels had in their time"].[1] This success was not limited to France: translated versions of her novels also appeared in English, Dutch, Romanian, Croatian, Italian, Spanish, and Portuguese.[2] After her death, fourteen editions of her complete works were published in France between 1817 and 1856, and translations of selected works were being published for her American reading audience as late as 1916.

In spite of this evident popularity, Cottin's novels have received little critical attention in either Europe or America since the mid-nineteenth century. Early twentieth-century assessments of her works as "inferior" by critics such as André Le Breton served to dissuade serious scholarship on Cottin for many years.[3] Leslie C. Sykes's *Madame Cottin*, published in 1949, was the only twentieth-century book-length scholarly study devoted exclusively to her life and works.[4] In the years since the publication of Sykes's book, an occasional journal article has attempted to draw attention to Cottin without, it appears, reviving any sustained scholarly interest in her.[5] Most likely as a consequence of feminist criticism's emphasis on rewriting/righting the canon, her name has begun to appear with greater frequency in recent literary histories, grouped with other women writers of her period.[6] However, the crucial connection between Cottin's self-perceived "defectiveness" and her literary production has yet to receive the critical attention it deserves.

For Sophie Cottin was a barren woman. Her correspondence reveals that she suffered from persistent amenorrhea—the absence of menstruation—throughout almost all of her mature life. Married in 1789 at the age of nineteen, she found herself widowed and childless four years later. As a result of many factors, including the writings of Jean-Jacques Rousseau, late-eighteenth-century France had become a fiercely pronatalistic culture, valorizing women essentially through their fertility, that is, through maternal production. Having openly espoused Rousseau's ideas on the proper social roles for women, Cottin understood well that there was little use for barren women like herself in postrevolutionary French culture. Caught between the ideological positions she had embraced and the reality of her sterility, she cast about for alternatives. Because of her cousin and best friend Julie Vénès Verdier's unique family situation, Cottin was allowed to become a permanent part of Julie's household and a sort of "second mother" to Julie's three daughters, a role that gave her great satisfaction. Though she never lacked suitors, she consistently resisted remarriage. Only in 1803, at the age of thirty-three, when—for a brief, miraculous moment—menstruation returned, did she allow herself to think once more that she could accept a marriage proposal. Shortly thereafter, when the obvious marker of fertility disappeared once again, she found herself forced to reveal her "defectiveness" to the man she had hoped to marry, and the relationship fell apart. She would die in 1807 at thirty-seven years of age, a childless widow.

In the early years of her widowhood, Sophie Cottin took up writing in a serious way and, as noted above, became one of the most successful novelists of her time. She admitted to finding writing therapeutic. I am convinced it was. Drawing upon modern research on infertility and its effects on human behavior, the following study of Cottin's five major works proposes that her writing bears the discernable traces of one barren woman's struggle, embedded in a culture that assigned her little or no value, to give meaning and purpose to her life. As psychologists Judith Daniluk, Arthur Leader, and Patrick J. Taylor have pointed out, "The infertility experience deals with the very essence of male and female sexuality and identity and thus may threaten a man or woman's basic concept of their masculinity or femininity."[7] Another researcher in the field, Jane Read, adds: "The issues that face those with a fertility problem may include fear that they are 'abnormal.' Many experience a loss of self esteem as well as a sense that they are not in control of the direction of their lives. They may face an existential anxiety, asking themselves questions regarding the purpose of their lives."[8] Sophie Cottin's fiction appears to wrestle with many of these anxieties and to seek an acceptable resolution.

My study begins with an overview of Cottin's early life during which, as her correspondence discloses, she formulated very definite ideas on gender roles. These ideas, however, eventually underwent a serious reevaluation when it became apparent to Cottin that motherhood, the only acceptable function for women in Rousseau's ideological system, was not in her future. An analysis of her first novel, *Claire d'Albe*, published anonymously in 1799, uncovers Cottin's revolt against the dominant discourse of her time regarding the measure of a woman's worth. The novels immediately following *Claire*, *Malvina* (1801) and *Amélie Mansfield* (1803), indicate that, for a significant period of time, Cottin wavered between open rebellion against and quiet submission to the prevailing cultural paradigm; as her reputation and her reading public grew, however, it appears that Cottin became increasingly convinced of her duty as a woman novelist to reinforce rather than reject the Rousseauian model. The heroines of her last two novels, *Mathilde* (1805) and *Elisabeth* (1806), accordingly perform their filial duties in spite of formidable opposition and suffering, confirming their allegiance to Father's law. Cottin died shortly after *Elisabeth* was published. We can only speculate on the direction subsequent writings may have taken, but it seems that the increasing religious devotion that marked the final years of her life would have continued to dominate her literary production.

There may have been good reasons why Leslie Sykes passed over Sophie Cottin's infertility as a minor detail. Perhaps in 1949, the year his book was published, such subjects were considered taboo. Perhaps in his own mind it carried little weight. Whatever his reasons, it left something essential yet to do in the analysis of Cottin's works, a critical lacuna that I hope to fill through the present study.

I am nevertheless deeply indebted to Sykes for his invaluable contribution to scholarship on Cottin. Working with descendants of the Cottin family line in the late 1930s, Sykes was able to compile and publish an impressive number of original letters, many of which had not previously been made available to the reading public. In some instances, he closed gaps in the historical record through the family's collective memory, among them the actual cause of Sophie Cottin's death, a subject of considerable speculation among previous biographers. In the end, Sykes's book was published by Basil, Blackwell, and Mott, a British firm, but nevertheless entirely in French, an indication of Sykes's enduring hope that French literati would find their way back to Sophie Cottin even if they had to pass through Oxford to get there.

Sykes's meticulous transcription of hundreds of letters—the great majority composed by Sophie Cottin herself but also including many others from her various correspondents—has been of immense value to my own work. Sophie Cottin had little formal education and, as a consequence, her letters are challenging reading in the original, filled as they are with misspellings and grammatical errors. Sykes eliminates most of these errors in his compilation of the correspondence, a practice that may make some historians squirm but also makes the actual reading decidedly easier. I pay tribute to his patience, a virtue I greatly admire.

I am aware of the fact that, due to the unavailability of Cottin's novels, any analysis of them must include a generous amount of plot summary if this study is to be of any use to my readers. I have therefore tried to strike a balance between description and interpretation. To those few who are already familiar with Cottin's oeuvre, I apologize in advance; my aim here is to engage all readers, initiated and uninitiated, in a new exploration of these works, and the study has taken its form from that fundamental consideration. In an effort to make this information available to as wide an audience as possible, I have provided English translations for all passages cited in the original French. I take full credit or blame for the results.

1
The Early Life of Sophie Cottin

ON 22 MARCH 1770, ANNE LECOURT, WIFE OF JACQUES RISTEAU, GAVE birth to her second daughter. The newborn was baptized the following day in St. Eustache Church, in Paris, and given the name Marie, to which her paternal grandmother, in her role as godmother to the child, added the name Sophie. Although the Risteaus were Protestants, French law required them to have their children baptized by a Catholic priest in order for the children to be officially recognized as citizens. The Catholic name Marie was quickly forgotten, the child thereafter called only by the name of Sophie.

The Risteaus were living in Paris at the time of Sophie's birth because her father was director of the prestigious Compagnie des Indes, having been named to that position in 1765. The Risteau family, however, were natives of Bordeaux, where they had established a reputation—and a fortune—as competent and trustworthy naval outfitters; Jacques, while still a young man, had been commissioned by Louis XV to build and arm four royal vessels. His success earned him the protection of M. d'Hérouville, commandant of Guyenne, who then orchestrated Jacques's appointment as director of the India Company. The Risteau family fortune evidently continued to increase as a result of this new position.

Two months after the birth of Sophie, according to family sources, at the death of his father, Jacques Risteau left Paris and returned with his family to Bordeaux, where most likely he assumed leadership of the family's shipwright business. In the absence of reliable records, we are left to imagine what Sophie Risteau's early childhood was like. We do know that she often vacationed at Bousquet, her maternal grandmother's property near Tonneins, where Sophie and her cousin, Julie Vénès, met and became lifelong friends and confidantes. As for her education, there is disagreement among her biographers: the frequent spelling errors in her correspondence have led some, like Marquiset, Quérard, and Lacoste, to refer to her education as "neglected" (*MC*, 4). Sykes, on the other hand, argues that, although evidently not the beneficiary of a structured classical education, she nevertheless shows signs in her earliest correspondence of a certain ease of expression, proof enough for him to side with Joseph Michaud in maintaining that Sophie's mother, a very cultivated woman, had taken considerable interest in educating her daughter. We do know for certain that Sophie had read Rousseau long before her marriage and, like many in Bordelaise society of the time, had become an avowed disciple.

There is no doubt that the single most important influence on Sophie Cottin's conception of female identity was the philosophy of Jean-Jacques Rousseau.[1] Cottin openly admitted to being persuaded by his arguments, particularly those found in *Emile* (1762), which she studied carefully. She could not have assimilated his ideas on children and education without at the same time confronting Rousseau's famous definition of woman's role in society:

> De la bonne constitution des mères dépend d'abord celle des enfants; du soin des femmes dépend la première éducation des hommes; des femmes dépendent encore leurs moeurs, leurs passions, leurs goûts, leurs plaisirs, leur bonheur même. Ainsi toute l'éducation des femmes doit être relative aux hommes. Leur plaire, leur être utiles, se faire aimer et honorer d'eux, les élever jeunes, les soigner grands, les conseiller, les consoler, leur rendre la vie agréable et douce: voilà les devoirs des femmes dans tous les temps, et ce qu'on doit leur apprendre dès leur enfance. Tant qu'on ne remontera pas à ce principe, on s'écartera du but, et tous les préceptes qu'on leur donnera ne serviront de rien pour leur bonheur ni pour le nôtre.

> [A child's health depends on the sturdy health of its mother; a man's primary education depends on the nurturing women give him; men's behavior, their passions, their tastes, their pleasures, their very happiness depend also on women. Thus women's entire education should be related to men. To please them, to be useful to them, to make themselves loved and honored by them, to raise them when they are young, to take care of them when they are older, to advise them, to console them, to make life pleasant and sweet for them: these are women's duties for all time and which should be taught them from childhood. If we do not return to this principle, we will not achieve our goal, and all the teachings they receive will do nothing either for their happiness or for our own.][2]

Woman's role thus centered on her destiny as mother, summed up by Rousseau in another notable passage:

> Les femmes, dites-vous, ne font pas toujours des enfants! Non, mais leur destination propre est d'en faire. Quoi! parce qu'il y a dans l'univers une centaine de grandes villes où les femmes, vivant dans la licence, font peu d'enfants, vous prétendez que l'état des femmes est d'en faire peu! Et que deviendraient vos villes, si les campagnes éloignées, où les femmes vivent plus simplement et plus chastement, ne réparaient la stérilité des dames? Dans combien de provinces les femmes qui n'ont fait que quatre ou cinq enfants passent pour peu fécondes! Enfin, que telle ou telle femme fasse peu d'enfants, qu'importe? L'état de la femme est-il moins d'être mère? et n'est-ce pas par des lois générales que la nature et les moeurs doivent pourvoir à cet état?

> [Women, you tell me, don't always have children! No, but their proper destiny is to have them. What! because there are in the world a hundred or so large towns in which women, living without moral principles, have few children, you maintain that the role of women is to have few! And what would your cities become, if the rural areas, where women live more simply and more chastely, did not compensate for the sterility of noblewomen? In how many provinces are women who have only four or five children considered infertile! In the end, what does it matter that such and such a woman has a small number of children? Is woman's role to be a mother lessened by that? and shouldn't nature and cultural practices support this role through universal laws?][3]

Rousseau reinforced this precept later in *Emile* in the section outlining the instructional program he called his "catechism for girls." Parodying the method employed by priests to teach children the doctrines of the church before their first communion, Rousseau substitutes the family servant for the priest and gives her the task of helping the daughters in the family memorize the right answers to questions concerning a little girl's expected future role in society:

> *La Bonne.* Et que deviennent les grandes filles?
> *La Petite.* Elles deviennent femmes.
> La Bonne. Et que deviennent les femmes?
> *La Petite.* Elles deviennent mères.

> [*Maid.* And what do big girls grow up to be?
> *Little Girl.* They become wives.
> *Maid.* And what do wives become?
> *Little Girl.* They become mothers.][4]

As Jean Elshtain explains, Rousseau's notion of female predestination to maternity based on biological "difference" followed quite logically from his theory on the evolution of human society: "Rousseau argues that sex distinctions arise and occur in nature prior to the pressures of civilization. Within the epoch of savage society, men and women established a division of labor that made biological sense given their respective reproductive roles. It was actual sex distinctions, then, occurring in nature, that set the basis for later socially constituted and buttressed distinctions. Distinctions between the sexes, both social and natural, are not for Rousseau 'the result of mere prejudice, but of reason.' Emile's and Sophie's education is, then, 'natural': it builds on a biological base; it is anchored in centuries of historic tradition; and it is morally preferable as the best means to preserve the public and private spheres alike."[5]

The concept of woman's predestination as mother, presented so self-assuredly by Rousseau, received a powerful boost from contemporary scientific discourse, as Yvonne Knibiehler has pointed out.[6] Typical of the kinds of medical and scientific texts that had tremendous influence in the late eighteenth century was Pierre Roussel's *Système physique et moral de la femme*. First published in 1775, this extremely popular and influential medical reader was reedited five times between 1775 and 1809. In it readers could find elements borrowed from three domains of knowledge that had remained separate up to that point: the field of the naturalists, because Roussel was a doctor and saw in woman *la femelle de l'homme*; the social domain begun by Rousseau, who defined woman by her role in society as wife and mother; and finally the field of the *moralistes*, who included among others Jean de Meung, Montaigne, La Rochefoucauld, and Molière. Roussel's system, for the first time, spoke of a *nature féminine*, total and separate from man's, and emphasized *la spécificité féminine*. Roussel's discourse refers more often to authority than to observed facts; he quotes Rousseau abundantly, for instance, especially book 5 of *Emile*, in which Rousseau's educational program for girls is outlined.

Knibiehler classifies Roussel as a *finaliste* because of his insistence that woman's body, by the presence of particular physical characteristics, destines her to a predetermined end, or *fin*. These physical characteristics are essentially two: frailty—*la faiblesse*—and the predestination to maternity. Woman's *faiblesse* condemns her to a life of passivity, characterized by limited activity and concentration on the life of the interior. Woman, however, can find consolation for this weakness in the idea of her beauty, but here again beauty is considered relative. Roussel maintains that a beautiful woman is a woman whose health and radiance promise fertility. Beauty is thus only a ruse of nature to achieve her ends.

The womb or uterus is the organ that attributes *spécificité féminine* to the woman more than any other, proving, as Roussel contends, woman's evident predestination for maternity. Knibiehler summarizes the argument: "Il y a chez la femme collusion étroite entre le physique et le moral, plus encore que chez l'homme: *tota mulier in utero*, répètent la plupart des auteurs après Hippocrate" ["There is in the female a strict collusion between the physical and the moral, more than for the male: *tota mulier in utero* [all of woman is in the womb], the majority of authors after Hippocrates have repeated"].[7] The *Encyclopédie* corroborated this stand: "la destination de la femme est d'avoir des enfants et de les nourrir" ["woman's destiny is to have children and to nurture them"].[8] The body of woman is suited for maternity; from the fact that she can be a mother, the rationalism of the time concluded that she must be one. Virey, a disciple of Roussel, followed up in his *Dictionnaire des sciences médicales* (1812–22) with this succinct definition of woman's role: "L'existence de la femme n'est qu'une fraction de celle de l'homme. Elle ne vit pas pour elle-même, mais pour la multiplication de l'espèce, conjointement avec l'homme. Voilà le seul but que la Nature, la Société et la Morale avouent" ["Woman's existence is but a fraction of man's. She lives not for herself but for the multiplication of the species, along with man. This is the only purpose that Nature, Society, and Moral Philosophy acknowledge"].[9]

Evidence of the widespread popularity of Rousseau's ideas on motherhood can also be found in French visual arts of the last half of the eighteenth century, as artists began increasingly to portray scenes of blissful domesticity and conjugal love, subjects that art historian Carol Duncan has sardonically labeled "new ideas in French art."[10] As Duncan points out: "After at least two centuries of ridicule, marriage began to enjoy a degree of popularity. Enlightened thinkers . . . almost unanimously regarded marriage as the happiest, the most civilized and the most natural of states, the institution that could best satisfy and conciliate social and individual needs. They generally agreed that in the marital relationship husbands should have final authority, but they also believed that only relationships based on mutual consent could work. To the material interests of the family they opposed the rights of the individual to personal happiness.... The promotion of these new ideas—the idea of childhood as a unique phase of human growth and that of the family as an intimate and harmonious social unit—became a major activity, a veritable cause, of Enlightenment writers."[11] Commissioned portraits of real families increasingly reflected these revitalized concepts, and it became fashionable even for women of noble rank to have themselves painted as mothers and wives.[12]

Greuze, who became Diderot's favorite painter, specialized in family and small village scenes with a heavy moralistic edge. His art, wrote Diderot, is "dramatic poetry that touches our feelings, instructs us, improves us and invites us to virtuous action."[13] Greuze's *Beloved Mother,* for instance, was one of the most popular attractions of the Salon of 1765. Duncan, in analyzing the painting, concludes that it "emphatically states that domestic life is blissful; it examines the very emotions of family relationships themselves, namely, the joy of being a husband and father and the delicious contentment of being a mother so well beloved by her husband and six children.[14] As in many such paintings he executed, Greuze emphasized the sensuality of the mother figure, who attracts the male through both her domesticity and her physical beauty. Of this painting, Diderot would write: "It says to all men of feeling and sensibility: 'Keep your family comfortable; ... [g]ive [your wife] as many children as you can ... and be assured of being happy at home.' "[15]

Jean-Honoré Fragonard who, like Boucher, had built his early reputation on erotic subject matter, turned to producing domestic scenes later in his career, most of them with a mother at the center of domestic activity, surrounded by children. One of the best examples of these is his *Heureuse fécondité (Happy Fertility)* (c. 1776–77), in which a young mother, holding a half-naked child in her arms, occupies center stage in a rustic country house setting. These two central figures look toward an open window, where a young husband leans looking in with obvious rapture on his face; he is accompanied by a donkey, to which one of the older children in the household offers a handful of hay. Two other small children sit on the floor at the side and knees of the young mother, while another woman, a servant or perhaps a relative of the mother, appears to be fending off the demands of a fifth child. The young mother's face and skin are milky white with rose highlights, matching perfectly the skin tones of the baby she holds. These two are the brightest objects on the canvas and are surrounded by warm tones of red, gold, and various shades of brown.

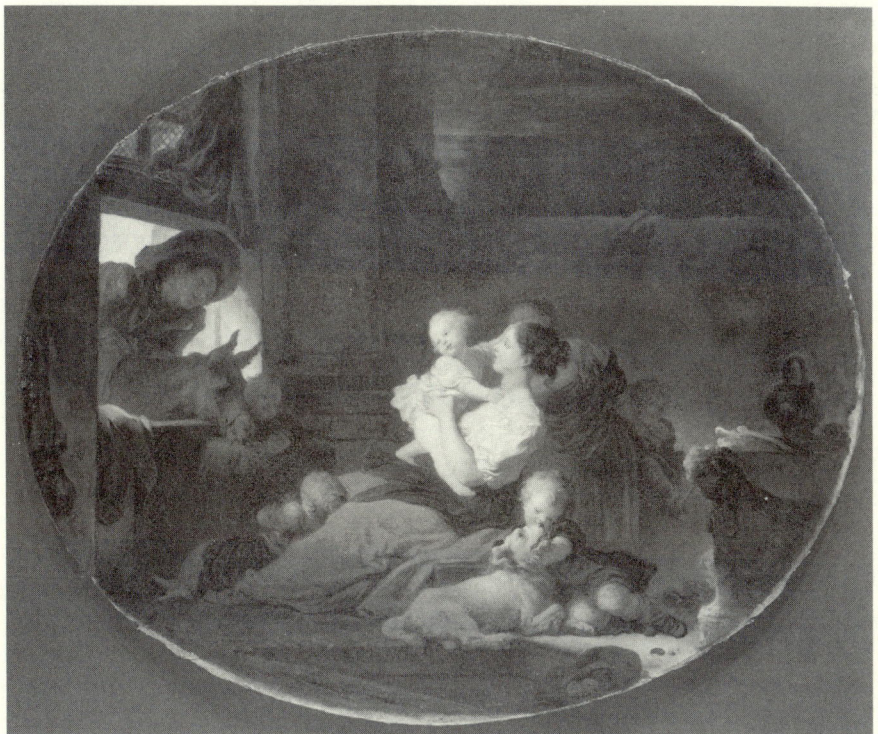

Fragonard, Jean-Honoré, *Heureuse Fécondité (Happy Fertility or The Happy Family)*, Timken Collection, Photograph © 2001 Board of Trustees, National Gallery of Art, Washington, after 1769, oil on canvas, oval; .539 × .651 (21¼ × 25⅝ in.).

The mother and child are illuminated by the light from the window, to be sure, but more importantly, they are lit up symbolically by the gaze of the young husband and father, whose countenance radiates love and admiration for the lovely, youthful mother of his offspring. He contemplates from his station—the exteriorized male public sphere—the interiorized and domesticized female, illustrating very neatly the "separate spheres" doctrine Rousseau had taught.

These dominant ideas defining female functions and social roles no doubt guided Sophie Risteau's mother in the education of her daughter. There would have been some training in literature but not enough to make of Sophie a *femme savante*. Emphasis would have been given to the practical arts—that is, domestic and homemaking skills—as well as to the refinement of the "pleasing arts" such as painting, drawing, and music. Sophie, like her counterpart in *Emile*, would have been trained especially to be a fit companion for a future husband.

In 1788, when Sophie was eighteen years old, she became engaged to Jean-Paul-Marie Cottin, who bore the title "squire," signifying a young nobleman who has not yet been named a chevalier. Cottin was seven years older than Sophie; his family was also Protestant. His grandfather had been the director of the India Company and ennobled in 1764. Cottin, like his father, was a banker. In the summer of 1788, he had come to Bordeaux on business and evidently to find a wife among the eligible Bordelaises. His first impression of Sophie Risteau was not favorable; describing her in a letter to his brother-in-law, he wrote: "La voix publique est en sa faveur, mais, je le répète, l'extérieur n'est rien moins qu'intéressant. Pas la moindre grâce, grande et maigre, laide, pas l'ombre de fraîcheur. . . . Comme elle est très timide, elle parle peu, et l'on ne peut juger de son esprit; cependant on dit qu'elle en a" ["Public opinion is in her favor but, I repeat, the outward appearance is nothing more than just interesting. Not a bit of grace, tall and thin, ugly, not the least trace of freshness. . . . Because she's shy, she says little, and one cannot evaluate her mind; yet others say she is intelligent"] (*MC*, 268).[16] Cottin apparently had a radical change of heart, however, as Sophie Risteau soon became the object of his undivided attention. On her part, she found it difficult to see herself as the object of a professed passion: "Je [me] trouve franchement si peu faite pour cela, que quand même je vois des preuves, je ne peux pas encore me persuader que ce soit possible" ["I find [myself] so poorly made for this that even when I see the proof, I still cannot bring myself to believe that it is possible"] (268). In their private conversations, words did not come easily to Sophie. And yet she found her affection growing for the young Cottin who, she was convinced, possessed "toutes les qualités précieuses et qu'il est si rare de trouver dans les jeunes gens d'aujourd'hui"["all the refined qualities, so rare in young men of today"] (269). Before long a marriage proposal was offered and accepted. It was decided that the marriage would take place in Paris and so on 17 October 1788, Sophie and her parents left Bordeaux, arriving at the Cottin family property in Guibeville on 23 October, when they met the future bridegroom's family. Sophie admitted to almost fainting from fright at the thought of the encounter, a situation that was most likely aggravated by the absence of her fiancé, who had been detained in Paris by business matters. Nevertheless, all signs seemed to predict a perfect alliance; as Sophie's mother claimed in a letter to her own mother, "fortune, état, considération, goût, caractère" ["fortune, status, esteem, taste, character"]—indeed, everything—pointed to an ideal match (270).

Health problems, however, delayed the marriage: Cottin fell ill with an intestinal disorder and the marriage was put off for six months while he convalesced. The Risteaus decided to stay in Paris and took up residence at the Hôtel de Chine on the rue de Richelieu. While there, Cottin's father began spitting up blood, a symptom of the tuberculosis that would kill him some five years later. Sophie kept herself busy with drawing lessons, music sessions with friends, embroidery, reading, and an occasional play. And of course there were the evening dinner parties at the Cottins' large home on the chaussée d'Antin, which Sophie usually found extremely boring.

All these details are recorded in the letters Sophie sent to her cousin and best friend, Julie Vénès–who would later become Julie Verdier through marriage—who had not accompanied the wedding party to Paris (*MC*, 271, n. 1). In letters to Julie from this period, Sophie claimed that her thoughts never strayed from her future husband, that everything she did now was centered on him: "Je trouvais cela ridicule dans les romans, et à présent je fais de même, non seulement sans y penser, mais malgré moi" ["I found this laughable in novels and now I am doing the same thing, not only without thinking but in spite of myself"] (272). Her evenings with Mme. Jauge, her fiancé's sister, allowed her to develop an admiration for this woman who, having married a man whom she did not love and who did not deserve her, had nevertheless molded her husband into an acceptable human being: "C'est elle qui l'a formé, qui l'a rendu ce qu'il est, c'est-à-dire très bien" ["She is the one who has educated him, who has turned him into what he is, that is, a good person"] (272). Sophie was obviously thinking about the power a woman could wield in marriage. Her marriage, she maintained, would be based on something more than love:

> Je ne veux absolument pas que tu donnes le nom d'amour à ce que j'éprouve. L'idée que j'ai de ce sentiment est qu'il est prompt et court, il vient aussi vite qu'il s'en va. Je suis bien loin d'avoir senti cela; le sentiment que j'éprouve est venu lentement, s'est fortifié à mesure qu'il a vu que l'objet qui l'avait fait naître en était digne.... [J]amais je n'aurai d'amour; j'aime trop mon ami, il possède toute ma tendresse, mon existence tient à l'espoir de faire son bonheur en le partageant.

[I insist that you not call what I am feeling by the name of love. The idea I have of that emotion is that it is quickly born and of short duration, it comes as quickly as it goes. I am far from feeling that way; what I feel came slowly, grew stronger only as it saw that the person who had caused its birth was worthy of it.... [N]ever will I love; I like my friend too much, he is the focus of all my tenderness, my existence depends on the hope that I will bring him happiness and share it with him.] (272)

Although her future sister-in-law's invitations to the theater guaranteed that Sophie had plenty of distractions to keep her entertained, she confessed that life at home was much more to her liking: "Il y a bien peu d'endroits où je m'amuse autant, où je sois aussi contente que dans la maison; j'ai des occupations, des pensées qui m'amusent délicieusement" ["There are very few places where I enjoy myself as much, where I am as happy as when I am at home; there I do things and entertain thoughts that amuse me in a delightful way"] (*MC*, 272). Her apparent natural timidity and her obvious discomfort when placed in public situations would lend credence to this avowed preference for the controlled environment of home.

The letters Sophie wrote to Julie during the waiting period before her marriage are replete with her reflections on topics dear to the heart of the "age of Rousseau." She defends, for instance, the virtues of "sensitivity": "Je ne suis point de l'avis que, parce que la vive sensibilité rend difficile sur le vrai bonheur, cela empêche d'être heureux; elle vous donne moins de sujets de l'être, mais elle vous fait jouir bien délicieusement de ceux qu'elle fait goûter" ["I am not of the opinion that, because a keen sensitivity makes true happiness difficult, it prevents happiness; [a keen sensitivity] gives you fewer things to be happy about, but it causes you to enjoy in a delightful way those it allows you to taste"] (*MC*, 273). Going on, she maintained: "Une âme sensible peut seule connaître l'amitié, elle ne pourra s'attacher qu'à une amie aussi tendre qu'elle.... Les sentiments vifs et durables, partagés par ceux qui les inspirent, sont seuls la base du bonheur" ["A sensitive soul alone can know friendship, she can only attach herself to a friend as tender as herself.... Deep and lasting feelings, shared with those who inspire them, are the only basis for happiness"] (273–74).

One memorable evening, the Cottins and Risteaus gathered around a table to read a rare copy of Mme. de Staël's *Lettres sur le caractère et les ouvrages de J.-J. Rousseau,* which M. Jauge had been able to borrow for a few precious hours. Sophie listened to her future husband read; the emphasis he gave to certain words and the emotion with which he read certain passages convinced her that their spirits were united. This revealing moment seemed to portend a union of equals (*MC*, 277). She described her behavior during the reading to Julie: "J'écoutais, je sentais davantage; mon coeur faisait tout et mon esprit rien" ["I was listening, [but] more than that I was feeling; my heart was doing everything and my mind nothing"] (*MC*, 277). In the renewed enthusiasm for Rousseau that Staël's work inspired, the group decided to read a few letters from his *Héloïse*. One of those read was Julie's letter to Claire in which she describes their friendship; at some point in the reading, Cottin's father exclaimed, "Mais c'est Sophie et sa cousine!" ["Why, that's Sophie and her cousin!"] (277). Sophie reaffirmed to her cousin that their friendship was an important and valuable part of her life: "Tu sais que si tu n'étais pas heureuse, ton amie ne pourrait jamais l'être, c'est à toi que tient une partie de mon existence" ["You know that if you are not happy, your friend could never be, a part of my existence is connected to you"] (275).

Sophie Risteau was married to Jean-Paul-Marie Cottin on 16 May 1789, at the Swedish embassy in Paris; both parties being Protestant, a special dispensation by Louis XVI was necessary to have the marriage recognized. The couple took up residence in the rue St-Georges in Paris. In the months following her marriage, Cottin's letters talked often of Rousseau; she was rereading his books as primers for marriage and motherhood: "Je relis avec plaisir la *Nouvelle Héloïse*, mais seulement les derniers volumes. Je leur trouve un charme, une douceur qui me pénètrent. Je trouve dans la courte analyse que Julie fait de l'éducation de ses enfants beaucoup de choses utiles. . . . J'aime Rousseau: ses ouvrages, ce me semble, sont dictés par la vertu, et il y a trop de naturel et de sentiment pour que son coeur n'est [*sic*] pas autant travaillé que son imagination" ["I am rereading *La nouvelle Héloïse* with pleasure, but only the last volumes. I find in them a charm, a sweetness that penetrates me. I find many useful things in Julie's short analysis of her children's education. . . . I love Rousseau: his works appear to me to have been dictated by virtue, and there is too much naturalness and feeling for his heart not to have worked as much as his imagination"] (*MC*, 279). Cottin's mother sent a copy of the *Confessions* to Julie Verdier; Sophie was sure that Julie would be "enchanted by it"(279). She admitted to Julie that she had begun to write on education. If she developed any sort of manuscript, it has since been lost, but it is safe to assume that Rousseau's own treatise on education served as the model for her system:

> *Emile* nous a jetés dans des discussions si longues et si opiniâtres que nous avons résolu de le quitter. Je soutiens Rousseau comme je soutiendrais mon meilleur ami; il mérite bien ce titre, par le bien et le plaisir qu'il m'a faits, et je t'avertis que si ta Delphine [la fille de Julie] est élevée suivant mes principes, qu'à seize ans je suis sûre de la pureté de ses idées, de l'honnêteté, de la sensibilité de son coeur. Je n'hésiterais pas à t'engager de lui laisser lire la *Nouvelle Héloïse*, comme un des meilleurs traités de morale. S'il fut jamais un livre fait uniquement pour les gens vertueux, c'est celui-là. . . . Dans ce siècle, il ne faut pas fermer les yeux des jeunes personnes sur les dangers qui les environnent, mais les leur montrer pour les en garantir."

> [*Emile* has thrown us into such long and violent discussions that we have resolved to leave it alone. I defend Rousseau like I would defend my best friend; he is worthy of the title because of the good he has done me and the pleasure he has given me, and I promise you that if your Delphine [Julie's daughter] is raised according to my rules, at age sixteen I can guarantee the purity of her ideas, her moral rectitude, and the sensitivity of her heart. I wouldn't hesitate to make you promise to let her read *La nouvelle Héloïse* as one of the best moral treatises. If ever there was a book written solely for virtuous people, it is that one. . . . In our day, one must not keep young people from seeing the dangers surrounding them but rather show them these things so as to keep them safe from them.] (280–81)

She defends Rousseau's Sophie as "un très bon exemple, puisqu'il représente une femme luttant et triomphant du plus dangereux de ses ennemis" ["a very good example, because he shows a woman who struggles and triumphs over the most dangerous of her enemies"] (279–80). Emile, on the other hand, is an example of a rare kind of man, and Cottin suggests that a woman would be better off not needing "un être aussi parfait" ["a being as perfect as he"] (280). The woman who has the greatest chance of being happy and faithful in marriage is the highly sensitive woman; because she feels everything so intensely, the marriage of friendship—as opposed to a marriage of love—provides her with sufficient stimulation to safeguard her against looking elsewhere. In this, Cottin appears to be commenting obliquely on her own marriage but more importantly, I think, on the reality of most eighteenth-century marriages. This is not to say, however, she continues, that such a woman would not have at times feelings of regret at not having a happier union; in fact, she may even dream about such a possibility without offending virtue, but this does not translate into behavior that would jeopardize her happiness and reputation. After all, she says, "il n'existe pas de bonheur parfait sur la terre" ["there is no perfect happiness on earth"] (280). In these few lines, we can find traces of the basic plot elements of her own first novel, *Claire d'Albe*, several years away yet from actual publication but slowly developing as a potential subject in her mind.

There is no question that Cottin, in addition to her interest in educational treatises and such, also loved a good novel. Or *any* novel, for that matter, in that even the bad ones could be instructive: "J'aime à pleurer, à être attendrie; je trouve que ce sentiment qui fait verser de douces larmes est agréable, aussi j'aime les romans. Un bon roman me dédommagera de plusieurs mauvais; j'en lis beaucoup, cela ne me gâte point le goût. Je trouve que souvent cela m'instruit: les auteurs, en faisant parler l'amour, l'amitié, les différents sentiments qu'ils traitent, disent ce qu'ils pensent et tout ce qu'ils sentent" ["I like to cry, to be moved emotionally; I find enjoyable that feeling that makes tears flow, and so I like novels. One good novel will cancel out several bad ones for me; I read a lot of them, it doesn't spoil my judgment. I find that often I learn something: the authors, in giving voice to love, friendship, and the other feelings they describe, say what they think and everything they feel"] (*MC*, 280). The key ingredients to novelistic production she claims to admire here would eventually find their way into her own work.

We cannot proceed further in this study of Cottin's life without now turning our attention to the important political events that affected every soul living in Paris at this time in history. As a married woman, Cottin carried the name of a family ennobled under the ancien régime; her father-in-law as well as her husband were solid supporters of the nobility, members of the *club de Valois*, which numbered among its members such luminaries as Talleyrand, Lafayette, and Condorcet (*MC*, 12). The name Cottin also appeared on the membership list of the Club monarchique—also known as les Amis de la constitution monarchique—founded in 1790; although we cannot tell in this case exactly which of the two, father or son, was involved, it makes little difference. Both father and son were committed to retaining the king as head of state and when, after the king's attempt to escape France failed in June of 1791 and the political climate shifted rapidly in favor of the radicals, Cottin *fils* decided it was in his best interest to leave Paris. Even Sophie was kept in ignorance of his hiding place, if we are to believe her letters, although it is possible she took the precaution of feigning ignorance in order to avoid the unpleasant possibility of the correspondence being intercepted by the very radicals her husband was trying to elude. In her letters to her husband-in-hiding, Sophie begged him to reconsider playing the hero:

> Qu'un jeune homme qui veut faire son chemin, et qui n'a aucun lien, endure toutes ces fatigues, qu'il mette tout son plaisir à se sacrifier à sa patrie, c'est très bien; mais je crois qu'on se doit à ses amis avant tout. . . . Je sais bien que, si tout le monde raisonnait ainsi, il n'y aurait pas beaucoup de patriotisme, mais il ne faut pas se faire illusion. Nous ne sommes plus dans ces temps héroïques où un homme qui se sacrifiait à ses concitoyens en était adoré; les têtes sont montées, mais le coeur est froid. . . . Un événement arrive, toutes les têtes s'échauffent, l'effervescence se communique, mais, le moment d'enthousiasme passé, on se rendort jusqu'à ce qu'un nouvel incident retire de la léthargie. Je le répète, le patriotisme s'endort dans la tranquillité.
>
> [For a young man who has no family to undergo such privation and find satisfaction in sacrificing himself for his country, that is all well and good; but I believe a man has an obligation to his friends above all else. . . . I know that if everyone thought this way, there wouldn't be much patriotism, but we should not fool ourselves. We are no longer living in those heroic times when a man who sacrificed himself for his compatriots became an object of their veneration; heads may be hot [in our day], but hearts are cold. . . . Something happens, everyone gets excited, the excitement spreads, but once the moment of enthusiasm has passed, everyone goes back to sleep until some new event shakes them out of their lethargy. I repeat, peace puts patriotism to sleep.] (281–82)

The Cottins' political situation must have changed significantly, however, in spite of Sophie's view of things, for by the end of 1791, Cottin had left France for England and taken his wife with him. This first stay in England lasted only two or three months, their quick return to Paris most likely incited by a fear of having their properties confiscated by the revolutionaries.[17] By August 1792, the Cottins were once more on the move, this time to the south and Spain, where they resided for several months; in January 1793, they returned to Paris. Shortly after their arrival, they received news of the death of Sophie's father who, along with his wife and oldest daughter and her children, had emigrated to Bath, England, in September 1792. Sophie's mother and sister would remain in Bath until 1800, when their names were officially removed from the government's list of émigrés. As Chateaubriand once described his own experience in a similar situation, the Cottins had returned to a place they called home, but in their absence, history had redesigned the stage, changed the scenery, and replaced the actors; nothing would be the same again.

Sophie's husband had suffered from ill health before his marriage. Now, the constant pressure of defending his estate against the revolutionaries, the loss of loved ones, and the imprisonment of relatives who were also his business partners apparently contributed to an aggravation of his already weakened condition. On 12 September 1793, Jean-Paul-Marie Cottin, thirty years old, died, leaving his wife, herself only twenty-three years old, a childless widow.

At the death of her husband, Sophie left Paris for Champlan, a property her husband had acquired jointly with his brother-in-law and business partner, Antoine-Louis Girardot, in June 1793. The property at the time consisted of two hundred hectares and was situated on one side of the Yvette Valley, approximately twelve miles from Paris, on the road from Corbeil to Versailles, between Palaiseau and Longjumeau. The house on the property was simple, with a garden and terrace from which the property gently receded to the river Yvette.[18]

Cottin was deeply depressed, admittedly suicidal at times; in letters to her mother, she explained that, "sentant le besoin de me livrer à des méditations qui pouvaient seules me raffermir, j'ai quitté Paris pour me jeter dans une solitude absolue" ["feeling the need to turn to meditation which alone could strengthen me, I left Paris in order to place myself in complete isolation"] (*MC*, 286). Her cousin and closest friend, Julie Verdier, came from Bordeaux to help her through the crisis. Evidently, the combination of a beautiful refuge in the countryside and the consolation of a dear friend began to have a salutary effect on Cottin; by November, she could write to her mother: "Ma douleur s'adoucit, mes idées se consolident et ma santé se raffermit. . . . [Des] pensées grandes et élevées m'ont redonné de l'énergie" ["My pain is easier to bear, my thoughts are becoming clearer and my health is improving. . . . [G]reat and noble thoughts have given me my energy back"] (286). One of these "great and noble thoughts" appears to have been her belief in the constancy and order of the natural world she observed at Champlan:

> Que l'univers m'étonne, de combien de merveilles je me vois entourée! Je ne puis décider lequel est le plus admirable: ou de la beauté de l'ensemble, ou de la finesse des détails, ou de l'ordre de tous deux. Je suis éblouie de ce magnifique tableau, confondue par la puissance qui le créa, et pénétrée de la bonté qui m'y plaça avec la faculté de le comprendre, de l'admirer. Cette conception immense anéantit ma raison. Mais si je ne comprends pas, je sens, et cela me suffit. Au milieu de l'ordre constant de la nature, un sentiment inutile et sans but n'aurait pas germé dans tous les coeurs; et parce que l'objet de mon amour m'est caché, est-ce une preuve qu'il n'existe pas? . . . Et dans tous les cas, ne pouvons-nous pas dire que tout ce que nous chérissons dans nos semblables est aussi incompréhensible, aussi invisible que la divinité? . . . Non, l'homme a beau se dénaturer, il ne deviendra jamais athée.

> [How the universe astonishes me, how many wonders I see myself surrounded by. I cannot decide which is the most admirable: the beauty of the whole, or the delicacy of the details, or the order of both. I am overwhelmed by this magnificent tableau, dumbfounded by the power that created it, and penetrated by the goodness that placed me here with the ability to understand and admire it. This immense creation destroys my reasoning powers. But if I do not understand, I feel, and that is good enough for me. In the midst of Nature's order, a useless, purposeless thought would not have been born in every heart; and because the object of my love is hidden from me, is it proof that he does not exist? . . . And in any case, can we not say that everything we love in others is just as incomprehensible, just as invisible as divinity itself? . . . No, man tries in vain to lose touch with his natural self, he will never become an atheist.](287)

The overtones of Rousseauian thought are plain in this passage; rather than finding consolation in orthodox Christian theology, Cottin obviously preferred the deism of her age.

Evidently, she perceived Champlan as crucial to the recovery of her health and, with Julie acting as intermediary, Cottin expressed to Girardot her desire to buy out his share and become sole owner of the property. The legal negotiations took longer than anticipated to resolve, made harder by the fact that both parties involved were under suspicion of the authorities. In July 1794, her name joined that of her mother-in-law's on the list of *émigrés,* and seals were affixed to her possessions at Champlan shortly thereafter, signifying the state's seizure of the property.

The seals were eventually lifted in September, but acquisition of the property was still uncertain as late as November 1794, when we find Cottin, despairing of ever having Champlan to herself, writing to her friend Gramagnac to ask him to find her a suitable apartment in Paris (*MC*, 294). The sale was evidently completed by spring 1795, when she could write to Gramagnac: "L'indépendance et la paix, voilà les seuls biens où j'aspire; j'en jouis et je ne veux pas les risquer, quand même je le pourrais" ["Independence and peace, these are the only things I seek; I am enjoying them at present and do not want to risk losing them, even if I could"] (296).

Finances would be a constant worry for her after her husband's death. Her father's fortune (estimated at 1,500,000 francs), to which she would have fallen heir, was converted by the revolutionary government into promissary notes worth less than 100,000 francs in real terms (*MC*, 17). And there was little hope of recovering her husband's assets after the arrest and imprisonment of his banking partners. When in 1794 it looked like she would have to sell Champlan itself to survive, she put her late mother's diamonds on the auction block (294). Like many of her class during these years, Cottin found her loss of loved ones made doubly bitter by the persistent threat of total financial disenfranchisement.

In an apparent effort to compensate for these losses, Cottin invited those persons she cared most for in life to be a part of her little community at Champlan. Her cousin Julie was of course the most vital part of this group; she would remain her closest and dearest friend her entire life. Writing to Gramagnac, she would claim: "Ma Julie est la meilleure partie de moi-même, elle est plus que mon amie, elle était celle de celui que j'ai aimé. Ce souvenir ajoute chaque jour à ma tendresse pour elle; comme j'aime à me confondre avec elle, il me serait doux que mes amis ne nous distinguassent pas l'une de l'autre" ["My Julie is the better part of myself, she is more than my friend, she was the friend of him whom I loved. This memory adds each day to my tenderness for her; as I like to consider myself identical to her, it would give me pleasure to have my friends unable to tell us apart"] (*UO*, 102).

Julie's husband and two daughters, Delphine and Elisa, aged three and one, also came to live at Champlan. To this circle were soon added Julie's older sister Félicité, a widow, with her daughter, Agathe, eleven years old. Cottin's mother also came to Champlan toward the end of 1793 but died shortly thereafter, in January 1794. The Edenic seclusion of Champlan was invaded more than once, however, by the Revolution, as noted earlier. In addition to the seizure of Cottin's possessions in July 1794, M. Verdier was arrested and imprisoned at Versailles. His wife followed him there to plead his case, leaving her two little girls in the care of Cottin. The situation forced Cottin to face the demon of depression once more: "La nuit, la nuit la plus noire lorsqu'elle m'enveloppe d'épaisses ténèbres, est encore moins sombre que mon âme" ["The night, the blackest night, when it enshrouds me in its thickest shadows, is still brighter than my soul"] (*MC*, 288). Writing to Julie at Versailles, she claimed: "Je suis dans un tel état de fatigue, ma Julie, que chacun de mes mouvements sont [*sic*] autant d'efforts qui m'épuisent. Je m'assois sans repos, je m'assoupis sans sommeil, je travaille sans objet, je chante sans plaisir; j'ai beau varier mes occupations, je n'ai jamais qu'une seule sensation. . . . Oh! pourquoi le temps ne vole-t-il pas plus rapidement pour amener cette calme époque, si cependant je suis destinée à y arriver?" ["I am in such a state of fatigue, my dear Julie, that every movement I make is so much effort, it completely drains me. I sit without resting, I lie down without sleeping, I work without a reason, I sing without pleasure; I try in vain to vary my tasks, I always have but one feeling. . . . Oh! Why doesn't time fly faster to carry me to that moment of peace, if I am destined to arrive there?"] (289). Time would come to her rescue, however; writing to Julie a week later, she could say: "Depuis hier j'ai eu quelques éclairs de bien, je jette des regards furtifs sur de douces espérances. . . . Je suis mieux; mon coeur est toujours triste, mais au milieu de ma mélancolie, je te le répète, j'ai senti, un instant, que mon existence pourrait devenir plus que supportable" ["Since yesterday I have had a few positive glimmers, I cautiously entertain some hopeful thoughts. . . . I am better; my heart is still sad, but in the midst of my melancholy, I repeat, I felt, for an instant, that my existence could become more than merely bearable"] (290).

In November 1794, Cottin wrote to Gramagnac, requesting that he send her the most recent laws on adoption of children. The reason?

> C'est un sujet dont je m'occupe depuis longtemps avec mon amie [Julie]. Je désire qu'elle me donne entièrement un de ses enfants, je consacrerais mon temps, ma vie, à m'en occuper, il remplirait le vide de mon coeur, je placerais sur lui toutes mes affections, toutes mes pensées, sa vie deviendrait ma vie, son bonheur serait le mien. Quand on a vécu dans un autre, il est si dur de revenir à soi; je ne puis plus

aimer comme j'ai aimé, mon âme est fermée à jamais à ce sentiment doux et pénétrant qui m'a animée quelques instants, mais je puis chérir cet enfant, je puis m'oublier pour lui. . . . Oui, je crois être sûre de pouvoir devenir la mère de l'enfant de mon amie, je crois pouvoir remplir tous les devoirs que ce titre [de mère] m'impose, je suis sûre de mes sentiments actuels, je crois pouvoir répondre du reste de ma vie.

[It is a subject that Julie and I have discussed for a long time now. I want her to give me one of her children entirely, I would dedicate my time, my life, to taking care of her, she would fill the emptiness of my heart, I would center all my affection, all my thoughts, on her, her life would become my life, her happiness, mine. When one has lived for someone else, it is so hard to fall back on oneself alone; I can no longer love as I have loved in the past, my soul is forever closed off to that sweet, penetrating emotion that inspired me for a short time, but I can love this child, I can devote myself to her. . . . Yes, I'm sure I can become the mother of my friend's child, I believe I can fulfil all the duties that this title [of mother] imposes on me, I am certain of my present feelings, and I believe I can guarantee they will not change for the rest of my life.] (*UO*, 65–66)

This effort to adopt one of Julie's children evidently did not come to fruition, but it is obvious that Cottin regarded herself as an equal participant in the mothering process. When Julie gave birth to her third daughter, Mathilde, in August 1794, Cottin announced in a letter: "Enfin nous voilà mères d'une troisième fille. Je ne m'afflige point de leur sexe, toutes les situations ont leurs jouissances, et une femme, quoi qu'elle en dise, peut être une créature heureuse; elle peut souffrir aussi beaucoup. Oui, personne le sait mieux que moi; mais cette peine n'appartient pas seulement à mon sexe, elle est l'apanage de tous ceux qui savent aimer, et malgré tout, qui voudrait renoncer à aimer?" ["At last, we are the mothers of a third daughter. I don't worry about their gender, everything has its good side, and a woman, in spite of what she says, can be a happy creature; she can also suffer greatly. Yes, no one knows this better than I; but this woe does not belong to my sex alone, it is the burden of all those who know how to love, and despite everything, who would want to renounce loving?"] (*UO*, 75–76).

Julie Verdier referred to Cottin as "l'amie qui sait toujours remplacer la plus tendre des mères" ["the friend who always knows how to stand in for the tenderest of mothers"] (*UO*, 78). This is corroborated by an incident described in Cottin's correspondence that reveals that she learned to play the surrogate mother role to perfection in caring for the children, making it virtually impossible for a stranger to distinguish between the biological and adoptive mothers through mere observation. In her letter, Cottin reports the visit of a young man new to the household, Jacques Lafargue, who watched as she dressed one of the children:

Je continue à m'occuper de mon enfant: Elisa était charmante en ce moment, elle m'a embrassée d'un air si tendre que son action est remarquée par cet homme, et il fait, non pas un compliment, mais une réflexion sur ce qu'il n'y a que la nature qui peut ainsi attacher un enfant à sa mère. Je souris et ne dis rien, il s'en aperçoit et me le demande. —C'est, lui dis-je, que vous faites en ce moment trop d'honneur à la nature, et que votre confiance en elle n'est qu'une erreur. —Comment! ne seriez-vous pas la mère de cet enfant? Oh! je ne veux pas le croire, je serais désolé. —Monsieur, pour la première fois que je vous vois, je ne veux point porter un sentiment si fâcheux dans votre âme, je ne vous dirai rien. —Vous m'avez déjà assez dit, je comprends mon erreur, et je m'afflige qu'on puisse ainsi feindre la nature. —Si je la feignais vous ne vous y seriez pas trompé; vous avez cru la voir parce qu'en effet elle est dans mon coeur. —Vous avez donc, a-t-il interrompu avec vivacité, surpassé la nature, et pour être mieux qu'elle, vous avez rompu ses barrières. —Ce n'est pas cela encore, mais il est des situations isolées où le besoin d'attachement fait qu'on s'attache violemment aux liens qui nous restent.

[I continued caring for my child: Elisa was charming and kissed me in such a tender manner that her action was noticed by this man and he made not a compliment but a reflection on how only nature can attach a child to her mother like that. I smiled and said nothing, he noticed and asked me why. "It's just that you're giving nature too much honor here and your confidence in her is but an error."

"How so? Aren't you the mother of this child? Oh, I can't believe it, I'd be embarrassed."

"Sir, since this is the first time I have seen you, I don't want to cause you any pain, and I will say nothing."

"You've already said enough, I understand my mistake, and I'm disturbed that one can imitate nature so well."

"If I were imitating it, you would not have made the mistake; you believed you saw it because, in actuality, it is in my heart."

"You have then," he interrupted with great enthusiasm, "surpassed nature, and to be better than she, you have exceeded her limits."

"That's not quite so, there are rare cases where the need for attachment causes us to hold on tenaciously to those relationships that are left us."] (*MC*, 299)

The assumptions about "nature" in this exchange are revealing: the eighteenth-century male observer assumes that the reciprocal affection in evidence here is due to biological bonds, hence physical determinacy. He is upset when Cottin informs him she is not the biological mother, but she reassures him in his presuppositions by claiming that the affection demonstrated comes from a true emotion, one indigenous to the female heart. Her affection for the child resembles in every way "natural" maternal love because it is first and foremost female; she admits, however, that her case may be rare, caused by a peculiar "need for attachment," a possible oblique reference to both her widowhood and her infertility.

In a poem she wrote for Julie in May 1795, Cottin paid tribute to her cousin for coming to her aid after her husband's death: "Quand le malheur pesait sur moi / Ta main adoucit ma misère" ["When misfortune weighed on me / your hand eased my pain"]. The two succeeding lines, however, pointed to an equally important benefit of their friendship: "Et je tiens à présent de toi / Le bonheur d'être presque mère" ["And because of you, I now have / the joy of being almost a mother"] (*MC*, 405). This state of being "almost a mother" would influence many of Cottin's decisions over the next few years.

In early September 1794, M. Verdier was released from prison to rejoin his family. Evidently, however, the marriage was already in trouble; in November 1794, there were ugly scenes at the house and Cottin wrote to Gramagnac, asking that he come protect them from the man she described as "an insane and wicked man": "Nous sommes dans l'état le plus cruel. M. Verdier abuse de notre sexe, de notre âge, de notre faiblesse, pour nous traiter avec une indignité dont je n'avais pas idée. Nous ne savons que faire sans protecteur, sans guide, nous nous trouvons abandonnées à la colère d'un homme qui ne ménage rien, qui nous menace des dénonciations les plus calomnieuses" ["We are in the cruelest of situations. M. Verdier takes advantage of our sex, our age, our weakness, to treat us with a vileness I had never imagined. We do not know what to do without a protector, without a guide, we find ourselves at the mercy of the rage of a man who holds nothing back, who threatens us with the most slanderous statements"] (*UO*, 67, 69). Her fears dissipated with the departure of M. Verdier for Paris, but Cottin insisted: "Sa femme, ses enfants, ne peuvent suivre un tel homme" ["His wife, his children, cannot follow such a man"] (68). There was, in her opinion, only one solution: "aujourd'hui tout est rompu, il n'y a plus rien entre eux, et le divorce les rendra aussi étrangers l'un à l'autre qu'ils auraient dû l'être toujours" ["today everything is broken off, there is nothing remaining between them, and a divorce will make them as estranged from one another as they should have always been"] (68–69). Cottin was adamant about the split: "Il a répandu mille horreurs dans ma maison, il a empoisonné notre paix, il dégraderait la vertu même s'il pouvait l'être. Non jamais un tel être ne vivra près de moi, je croirais faire une chose mauvaise et coupable que d'y consentir, je veux que tout ce qui m'entoure soit pur et honnête" ["He has poured out a thousand afflictions on my household, he has disturbed our tranquillity, he would debase virtue itself if he could. No, never will such a person live near me, I would consider it a crime to consent to such a thing, I want everything around me to be pure and upright"] (69). Cottin was anxious to see Verdier return to his own home: "Il me tarde qu'il soit bien loin, il me tarde surtout que mon amie ait brisé tout à fait la chaîne qui lui a fait verser tant de larmes" ["I am anxious to see him a long way away, I am anxious especially that my friend completely break the chain that has caused her to shed so many tears"] (69).

Verdier did return to Tonneins, leaving his wife and children behind at Champlan, but, in spite of Cottin's wishes, he and Julie never formally divorced. Divorce had not always been a possibility for a woman in Julie's situation; it was only thanks to the Revolution that it had become so. Cottin seemed to be grateful for the chance a woman had to rectify a mistake made earlier in marrying the wrong man—in this case, a much older man whose behavior, evidently, was unacceptable. There was a way out now for a woman; she did not have to continue to live in misery, to suffer indefinitely, and Cottin appears to have recognized and appreciated the new option in these letters.

Verdier's departure did not leave the women without male companionship, however. On the contrary, Cottin was visited regularly by male friends. There was first of all Gramagnac himself, an old and trusted friend. Without his help, it is unlikely she would have survived the first two years of widowhood. Gramagnac became, next to Julie, Cottin's most valuable confidant during this time, entrusted with tasks both small and great. It was not long, however, before he began to imply more than just friendship in his letters and visits to her. Cottin was bothered by this; his interest in her as a candidate for marriage forced her to explain very clearly that she was not looking for a husband, that friendship was what she sought in male companionship. Explaining her feelings in a letter, she wrote: "La situation où je suis est la seule qui me convienne. L'indépendance et la paix, voilà les seuls bien où j'aspire; j'en jouis et je ne veux pas les risquer, quand même je le pourrais. . . . Il n'est aucun état dans la vie, aucune situation, qui puisse remplir l'idée du bonheur que je me fais" ["The situation I am in is the only one that suits me. Independence and peace, these are the only riches to which I aspire; I am enjoying them here and don't want to risk losing them, even if I could. . . . There is no condition in life, no situation that can measure up to the idea of happiness that I have for myself"] (*MC*, 296).

After the summer of 1795, Gramagnac seems to have disappeared from her life, most likely to pursue other options. He was only the first in a long line of suitors who courted Cottin unsuccessfully over the years. Perhaps the best known of the group, the one whose story appears to have held the most interest for Cottin's early biographers, was Jacques Lafargue, the son of Cottin's cousin Félicité. While Cottin's husband was alive, Jacques had visited the Cottins during their exile in Champlan and in August 1792 he accompanied the couple on their trip to Spain. He later enlisted in the republican army but was sent home because of illness; while on sick leave in September 1794, he came to live with his mother and the other women at Champlan. He was then eighteen years old, suffering from an inferiority complex and ennui, as he confessed in his autobiographical writings (*MC*, 27).

Cottin appears to have been drawn to him out of motherly instinct; he in turn was attracted to her because of her understanding and patience. Julie and others warned Cottin that things were getting more serious than she thought, but she simply shrugged it off. How could she ever consider a union with a child like Jacques? The idea was, she claimed, "monstrous"(*MC*, 28). She had to admit, though, that there was something beneficial, almost therapeutic, in Jacques's interest in her: "La perte de mon époux avait laissé un double vide dans mon coeur; je souffrais de ne plus rien aimer, je souffrais de ne plus être aimée. Mon imagination, sans doute exaltée par ce que je croyais devoir à sa mémoire, m'avait fait jurer de ne plus former de nouveaux liens; mais mon coeur, souffrant de ce serment téméraire, cherchait à se dédommager du veuvage que je lui imposais, en s'entourant de liens d'amitié" ["The loss of my husband had left a double void in my heart; I suffered from having nothing more to love, I suffered from no longer being loved. My imagination, undoubtedly excited by what I thought I owed to his memory, had made me swear never to develop a new relationship; but my heart, suffering from this rash vow, sought a way to alleviate the widowhood I had imposed on it, by surrounding itself with friendship"] (28).

During this time, Cottin continued to shun Parisian high society, preferring instead the intimate familial association with Julie and her daughters. In a letter addressed to Jacques Lafargue dated June 1795, she adamantly defended her conduct, claiming it was based on her concept of female duty and responsibility to the state:

> Le bien qu'une femme peut faire à son pays, ce n'est pas de s'occuper de ce qui s'y passe et de donner son avis sur ce qui s'y fait, mais de pratiquer dans son petit entourage le plus de vertus qu'elle peut, de tâcher d'y donner l'exemple des bonnes moeurs, de l'amour du travail, de s'y adonner aux occupations de son ressort, tels que les soins domestiques et l'éducation de ses enfants. Les femmes doivent se borner à faire le bien en détail, et leurs facultés ne peuvent guère s'étendre plus loin que leur petit monde; mais que chacune y remplisse bien ses devoirs, et de cette multitude de bonnes choses naîtra un ensemble bien ordonné. C'est aux hommes qu'appartiennent les grandes idées, c'est à eux à établir le gouvernement et les lois; c'est à nous à en faciliter l'exécution, en faisant ce que nous devons faire, et pas autre chose. Pour que tout aille bien, il faut que chaque partie reste à sa place; c'est pour ne pas être à la mienne que je manque de cette bienveillance universelle qui est assurément une des vertus essentielles de mon sexe. . . . C'est ainsi que, pour m'être écartée de la route que j'aurais dû suivre, j'ai perdu une vertu charmante; mais je veux la recouvrer, j'ai besoin de la sentir, je sais où je peux la trouver: c'est en revenant à ma place. Du moins n'en ai-je pas perdu le goût; au contraire, je sens qu'il me sera bien doux d'être encore tout ce que je peux être.

> [The best thing a woman can do for her country is not to get involved with what is going on or voice her opinion on what is happening, but to practice in her own circle the greatest virtues she can, to endeavor to give a good example of correct behavior and a love for work, to concentrate on her own pursuits such as domestic duties and her children's education. Women should limit themselves to doing good in the small things; their abilities can scarcely extend beyond their own little world; but let each one of them do her duties well and from this multitude of good things will be born a well-ordered whole. Great ideas belong to men; it is up to them to establish the government and

its laws; it is up to us to assist in their implementation, in doing what we should do and not something else. For everything to go well, each part should stay in its place; it is because I am not in my own that I lack that universal benevolence that is surely one of the essential virtues of my sex.... It is because I strayed from the path I should have followed that I lost a charming virtue; but I want to recover it, I need to feel it, I know where I can find it: it is by coming back to my place. At least I have not lost my desire for it; on the contrary, I feel that it will be very sweet to be once again everything I can be.] (*MC*, 301–2)

It appears that, over the course of two years of close contact and in spite of her initial resistance to the idea, she began to have feelings for the young man, but the possibility of marriage with Lafargue was never an option. When in June 1796 Lafargue was released from his military obligation, Cottin found a job for him in Paris. At first, Lafargue wrote regularly and returned to Champlan as often as possible to visit; then the frequency diminished gradually until Cottin no longer received anything from him. His health was reportedly deteriorating rapidly. She wrote to ask: "Votre peine vient-elle de cette résolution irrévocable de ne jamais m'unir à vous? Si cela est, dites-le moi; ... Je peux résister à tout, à votre amour, à ma tendresse, mais non pas à votre peine" ["Does your pain come from my irrevocable resolve never to marry you? If so, tell me; ... I can resist anything, your love, my tender feelings, but never your pain."] (*MC*, 29). What is interesting here is that she refers to his affection as love while hers is only tenderness; the maternal overtones are strong in this note.

Julie, sent to ascertain just how bad Lafargue really was, returned with the report that the doctor had predicted the boy would go mad if not treated immediately. Lafargue was consequently brought to Champlan for rehabilitation. He swore to Cottin that his passion for her had died; he treated her coldly. But Cottin knew something was wrong: "Tiens, Julie, ne dis cela à personne, mais j'ai trouvé dans ses yeux quelque chose de farouche" ["Listen, Julie, don't tell anyone, but I saw something wild in his eyes"] (*MC*, 301). On the night of 23 August 1796, while sitting in the orangery, Larfargue blew his brains out. Félicité, who considered Cottin responsible for her son's death, left Champlan, never to return and evidently never to forgive. These events caused Cottin to write:

Je n'en puis plus, la langueur m'accable, l'ennui me dévore, le dégoût me poursuit, je souffre sans pouvoir dire de quoi, le passé et l'avenir, les vérités et les chimères ne me présentent plus rien d'agréable. Je suis importune à moi-même, je voudrais fuir et ne puis me quitter; rien ne me distrait, toute occupation m'excède, les plaisirs ont perdu leur piquant et les devoirs leur importance. Je suis mal partout; si je marche, la fatigue me force à m'asseoir; quand je me repose, l'agitation m'oblige à marcher. Mon coeur n'a pas assez de place, il étouffe, il palpite violemment; je veux respirer, et de longs et profonds soupirs s'échappent de ma poitrine. Où est donc la verdure des arbres? Les oiseaux ne chantent plus. L'eau murmure-t-elle encore? Où est la fraîcheur? Où est l'air? Un feu brûlant court dans mes veines, je me consume, des larmes rares et amères baignent mes yeux et ne me soulagent pas. . . . [L]a verdure est morte dans la nature, comme l'espérance dans mon coeur. Dieu! que l'existence me pèse!

[I cannot go on, I am overcome by listlessness, anxiety is eating me up, I am hounded by loathing, I suffer without being able to say why, the past and the future, facts and fictions no longer offer me anything attractive. I am a vexation to myself, I want to run away and yet cannot flee myself; nothing amuses me, everything I do exasperates me, pleasures have lost their attraction and responsibilities their importance. I am unhappy everywhere; if I walk, weariness forces me to sit down; when I rest, anxiety forces me to get up and walk. My heart feels cramped, it suffocates, it beats violently; I want to breathe, and long, deep sighs escape from my breast. Where is the greenery of the trees? The birds no longer sing. Does the water still babble? Where is the coolness? Where is the air? A burning fire races in my veins, I am burning up, tears, rare and bitter, bathe my eyes and do not relieve me. . . . [N]ature's greenery is dead, like the hope in my heart. God! how life weighs on me!] (*MC*, 305)

Even the children became a burden in these moments: "Mes enfants, je pensais à vous alors, je n'y pense plus que pour être importunée de vos jeux et tyrannisée par la nécessité de vous rendre des soins. Je veux vous ôter d'auprès de moi, je veux en ôter tout le monde, je veux m'en ôter moi-même" ["My children, I used to think of you, now I think of you only as your games disturb me and the need to take care of you forces me. I want to get rid of you, I want to get rid of everyone, I want to get rid of myself"] (*MC*, 306). Nature, which had been so benevolent before, now became just another source of suffering: "Lorsque le jour paraît, je sens mon mal redoubler. Que d'instants comptés par la douleur! Le soleil se lève, brille sur toute la nature: il me flétrit et je me sens mourir, que je meurs d'un mal cruel, inconnu à moi-même" ["When the day dawns, I feel my pain redouble. So many moments counted in suffering! The sun rises, shines on all of nature: it wilts me and I feel myself dying, dying of a cruel sickness, a mystery to myself"] (306).

As Sykes points out, this letter had no particular addressee and thus sounds more like a journal entry than a letter; parts of it, quoted word for word, would actually find their way into her first novel, *Claire d'Albe*, implying—perhaps, though not definitely—that Cottin had the piece to refer to when she began writing her novel. Whatever the case may be, it is obvious that Champlan no longer held the same magic it once had for her. An invitation from relatives to share a house with them in Paris seemed at first to Cottin to offer the "peaceful and independent life" she now sought. Julie and the children would accompany her, they would set up their own "separate little household" on one of the floors of the spacious house, and Cottin's house would become "le temple . . . des arts et de la liberté" ["the temple . . . of the arts and of liberty"] (*MC*, 308). The move was made sometime in the autumn of 1796. Commenting on the break with the past the move symbolized, she wrote to Amable Pelet, friend of Lafargue: "Les trois années passées à Champlan se découperont sur le tissu de ma vie d'une manière tranchante; tout ce qui fut avant, tout ce qui sera après, ne leur ressemblera point; les fils qui l'ont formé sont tous brisés ou le seront bientôt, mon amie [Julie] seule me reste" ["The last three years in Champlan will stand out sharply against the fabric of my life; everything that came before, everything that comes after, will not match them; the threads that formed them are all broken or will soon be, only my friend [Julie] remains"] (307).

The death of Lafargue and the flight from Champlan appear to have thrown Cottin into a depression similar to that she had experienced after her husband's death, judging from another letter written to an unknown correspondent during this time: "A présent me voici arrivée à 25 ans, n'ayant presque connu des passions que les douleurs qu'elles causent et le vide qu'elles laissent. J'ai vu autour de moi les illusions s'écrouler, l'amour s'enfuir, et les espérances desséchées décolorer le reste de mon existence. . . . La tranquillité ne peut être appréciée par celui dont elle est l'état habituel: il faut avoir été déchiré par les anxiétés de la douleur, pour savoir combien il est doux de ne plus souffrir" ["Here I am twenty-five years old, having known only the suffering that passion can bring and the emptiness it leaves. I have seen my illusions crumble around me, love flee, and dried up hopes stain the rest of my life. . . . Peace cannot be appreciated by the person for whom it is a habitual condition: you have to have been torn apart by the anxieties of suffering, to know how sweet it is to no longer suffer"] (*MC*, 309). Continuing to count up her losses, she claimed: "A 25 ans, une femme peut continuer à aimer, mais elle ne recommence plus" ["At twenty-five years of age, a woman can continue to love, but she can't start all over again"] (309). Passion could perhaps give a few days of ecstasy but afterward, what price would one have to pay? No, she says, a woman of her age "doit veiller avec soin sur ce peu d'instants qui la séparent encore de l'âge du calme, afin d'empêcher qu'ils ne soient troublés par de nouvelles tempêtes. . . . Elle doit employer l'activité morale qui lui reste à se faire une vie douce, paisible et indépendante" ["should carefully protect the short period of time remaining before she enters the calm stage of life, to keep it from being disrupted by new storms. . . . She must use her remaining moral strength to create a calm, peaceful and independent life for herself"] (309).

Cottin, however, was not well suited to Parisian life. A very frank letter from Amable Pelet, her confidant during the Lafargue episode, gives us his assessment of both her qualities and her weaknesses, which seem to have condemned her never to fit in with the Parisian bon vivants:

> Le peu d'instants que j'ai passés auprès de vous m'a fait distinguer parfaitement toute la droiture de votre coeur, toute la bonté de votre caractère, et les défauts que vous avez. Ces défauts serviront encore à vous faire chérir de tous ceux qui vous aimeront, et à qui vous aurez seulement dit que vous les aimez; et vous avez en vous quelque chose que je ne puis expliquer, qui rendra ces défauts vénimeux pour les autres et bienfaisants pour vous. Ce que je vous dis là peut paraître extraordinaire, mais cela est exact, peut-être même le sentez-vous vous-même. Je ne crains pas de vous le dire, vous êtes une femme dangereuse à vous-même, par la facilité que vous avez à vous enthousiasmer pour le beau idéal, que vous ne trouverez pas plus que le bonheur parfait. Ce qui vous empêchera d'être nuisible aux jeunes gens du monde, c'est qu'ils ont des yeux qui ne font que voir et des sens qu'ils ne savent satisfaire que stupidement, et vous n'êtes point faite pour ces gens-là. Vous n'avez pas une jolie figure, mais vous avez une expression de physionomie qui gagne à être environnée de jolis visages. Vous n'avez pas une belle taille, ni un maintien de mode, mais votre démarche, vos manières sont tellement en rapport avec votre physionomie et votre son de voix, qu'on ne désire pas que vous soyez autrement et qu'on craint que vous ne changiez.

> [The few moments I spent in your presence allowed me to see perfectly the upright nature of your heart, all the generosity of your

character, and your weaknesses. These weaknesses will serve to make you dear to all those who love you and to whom you have merely expressed love; and you have something in you that I cannot explain, which will make these weaknesses poisonous to others and wholesome to you. What I am telling you here may seem extraordinary, but it is true, perhaps you even feel it yourself. I am not afraid to tell you, you are a danger to yourself, because of the ease with which you become excited about perfect beauty, which you will not find any more than you will find perfect happiness. What will save you from being destructive to the young men of the world is the fact that they have eyes that merely see and senses that they only know how to satisfy in ignorant ways, and you are not made for those kinds of people. You do not have a pretty face, but you have an expression that benefits from being surrounded by pretty faces. You do not have a pretty figure, or stylish dress, but your behavior, your actions are so much in harmony with your expression and the sound of your voice, that one doesn't desire you to be any other way and fears any change.] (*MC*, 309)

With this letter, Pelet returned Cottin's portrait and bid her adieu. It is not clear why exactly he broke off with her at this point. If the pattern we have seen in her actions after the death of her husband was repeated here, it simply meant that Pelet recognized that there was no hope of any relationship developing into marriage with her, hence the return of the portrait.

Is it possible, on the other hand, that Pelet was one of those young men he mentions in this letter who, looking for physical beauty only, cannot appreciate what a woman like Cottin offered? He seemed capable of seeing beyond the surface level, of appreciating the harmony that existed between Cottin's earnest, wholesome appearance and the uprightness of her character. But in the end, was she, because of her idealism, too dangerous for a man like himself? We can only wonder. Cottin described herself to Julie in a letter dated near this same time as one of those people "romanesques dans leurs sentiments, et exagérés dans la vertu" ["romantic in their feelings, and overzealous in their virtue"] (*MC*, 314). She admitted to being attracted to the new looser moral code of postrevolutionary Paris, mainly because of her natural *penchant*, but "qui pourrait changer des devoirs aussi enracinés, aussi chéris? . . . Cette honnêteté, qui a toujours été mon idole, se représente avec tous ses charmes, et quand je veux lui demander compte des plaisirs qu'elle m'a procurés, elle me présente le tableau des peines qu'elle m'a épargnées. —Nul remords, me dit-elle, n'est entré jusqu'à présent dans ton coeur, et tu ne peux imaginer combien ce bien que tu me dois est inappréciable" ["who could change such deeply rooted, such prized values? . . . This moral rectitude, which has always been my idol, presents herself with all her charms, and when I want to make her count up all the pleasures she has cost me, she shows me the picture of all the pain she has saved me. 'No remorse,' she tells me, 'has yet penetrated your heart, and you cannot imagine how invaluable this gift is that I have given you'"] (314–15).

Later, she described other reasons for her dissatisfaction with Parisian life: "Le séjour de Paris m'est pernicieux; je trouve que l'air qu'on y respire est comme un poison qui agite sans objet, qui émeut sans plaisir, qui répand le dégoût au dehors et l'ennui au dedans, mais c'est un ennui actif. . . . Suis-je avec des gens médiocres, je m'endors au murmure de leur nullité; suis-je dans un cercle de beaux esprits, la doublure déchire là-dessus, je ne vois que la prétention, et je me tais ou je persifle. . . . Je deviens moi-même le premier objet de ma critique. Ma vanité me semble misérable; ses tourments, ses efforts et ses victoires me font également rougir" ["Living in Paris is harmful to me; I find the air that one breathes here is like a poison that makes you agitated but without a reason, exciting you without giving pleasure, spreading disgust on the outside and boredom on the inside, but it's an active boredom. . . . If I'm with mediocre people, I fall asleep to the murmur of their droning; if I'm with a group of clever people, the veil tears away, I see only affectation and I fall silent or I mock them. . . . I am becoming the main subject of my own criticism. My vanity appears petty to me; its cares, its struggles, and its conquests all cause me to blush in shame"] (*MC*, 324–25).

Frankly summarizing her life, she declared: "Je suis veuve, je n'ai point d'enfants, je n'ai que 25 ans, et je ne vais jamais au bal. Cela me donne un loisir extrême; je l'emploie quelquefois à faire des vers, de peur de plus mal l'employer encore. Quand l'imagination travaille, le coeur repose, et dans le calcul, si la nature murmure, la prudence applaudit, et si le bonheur n'y trouve pas son compte, la tranquillité y trouve le sien" ["I am a widow, I have no children, I am only twenty-five years old, and I never go to parties. This gives me a lot of leisure time; I use it sometimes to write poetry, for fear of using it in some more useless way. When the imagination is at work, the heart rests, and in the end, if nature grumbles a bit, wisdom approves, and if happiness isn't fully satisfied by it, tranquility is"] (*MC*, 314). This passage from her correspondence of April 1797 is the first mention made of a writing project since her reference to the book on education begun in

1790. From this time on until her death in 1807, she would not cease writing. Had she reached a point in her life now where writing had become an imperative, an indispensable therapeutic exercise she could use to work through the problems detailed above?

During the summer of 1797, she was once again offered marriage, this time by Constant Lemarcis, another cousin who had been a widower for several years (*MC*, 33). He, like others before and after him, would be refused. Cottin persisted in staying by Julie and the children who, Sykes suggests, may have come to depend on her for financial security after Julie's separation from her husband (34). There may have been other, more important aspects here, in addition, as we see in her letter to Julie written in July 1797. In it, Cottin talks frankly of the realities of marriage in the eighteenth century; she is very aware that being a widow is perhaps the most powerful position she can have as a woman in her century, in that she controls her own property. And once again there is the question of the children:

> Je regarde mon amitié pour toi, et mon indépendance, attachées l'une à l'autre. En perdant cette dernière, en donnant à un être quelconque un droit sur mes actions, ma personne et ma fortune, je ne suis plus sûre de vivre avec toi, tes enfants ne sont plus les miens, mon sort est changé. Ce sort que je prévois m'est bien cher; il en est peu de plus heureux, et si je regarde tous les ménages qui m'entourent, je dis même qu'il n'en est point. . . . Nous ne sommes plus au temps des illusions, mon amie, il faut voir les choses telles qu'elles sont; et du moment qu'un homme aurait droit sur ma fortune, je ne serais plus maîtresse d'en faire l'usage que je voudrais. . . . Jamais, non jamais, je ne courrai un pareil risque: les devoirs de l'humanité, ceux mêmes de l'amitié, sont pour moi les plus sacrés de tous, et je ne veux pas qu'une volonté étrangère puisse jamais y mettre obstacle. . . . [C]omme je ne veux plus mettre la raison de personne à la place de la mienne, je ne veux rendre aucune volonté maîtresse de la mienne. Dans le mariage, loin d'être libre, on est observé; que je le veuille, que je l'approuve ou non, je suis obligée de céder. . . . C'est donc d'après tous les inconvénients, je dirai même les malheurs, attachés à l'état de mariage, que j'ai juré de ne jamais y entrer; et ce serment, je le tiendrai. . . . Oui, le devoir m'attache à toi et à tes enfants; je voudrais non seulement l'amitié, mais la protection et le dévouement. . . . Je tiens presque ton sort entre mes mains, j'y tiens peut-être celui de trois créatures innocentes et adorées; et je donnerais à un autre le droit de les protéger, je courrais la chance affreuse qu'il leur fît sentir le poids? . . . Idée affreuse!
>
> [I consider our friendship, and my independence, as linked one to the other. In losing the latter, in giving power over my actions, my person, and my fortune to someone else, I can no longer be assured of

living with you, your children will no longer be my own, my future is changed. This future I foresee is very dear to me; there are very few happier, and when I look at all the households around me, I can even say that there is none [happier].... We no longer live in the age of illusions, my friend, we must see things as they truly are; and as soon as a man got power over my money, I would no longer be able to do with it as I pleased.... Never, no, never, will I run such a risk: duty toward humanity, that even of friendship, is for me the most sacred duty of all, and I never want to allow an outsider's will to become an impediment to that.... [A]s I never again want to replace my own thought with that of someone else, I do not want to allow any other will to become the master of my own. In a marriage, far from being free, one is under scrutiny; whether I want it or not, whether I approve of it or not, I am forced to yield.... It is therefore because of the problems, I will even say the unhappiness, attached to the marriage state, that I have sworn never to enter into it; and this oath, I will hold to.... Yes, duty attaches me to you and to your children; not only friendship, but also protection and devotion.... I almost hold your fate in my hands, I hold perhaps that of three innocent and beloved creatures; and would I give another the right to protect them, while running the terrible risk that he would abuse that right?... What a horrible idea!] (315–17)

In a follow-up letter, she reiterated to Julie:

Je pense, comme toi, que l'état le plus heureux est celui d'un mariage assorti, mais il faut, pour y parvenir, une situation particulière, et celle-là n'existe et ne peut plus exister pour moi.... Pour que l'âme puisse toujours brûler d'amour, il faut qu'elle ait encore toute sa vie, toute sa vigueur, qu'elle n'ait point été flétrie par le malheur, ni éveillée par la crainte.... [Q]uand on a vécu, quand on a souffert, on peut encore peindre avec fraîcheur ce qu'on a senti, et non l'éprouver encore. Mon coeur, Julie, ne pourrait plus suffire au bonheur d'un mariage heureux.

[I think, as you do, that the happiest state is a harmonious marriage, but to achieve it, you need a certain situation and that does not exist and can no longer exist for me.... In order for the soul to burn with love still, it needs to have all its life yet, all its strength; it can't have been blighted by sorrow nor alarmed by fear.... [W]hen you've lived, when you've suffered, you can still vividly describe what you've felt, and yet not feel it anymore. My heart, Julie, could no longer furnish what it takes to achieve happiness in a happy marriage.] (317)

These arguments, persuasive in their own right and echoed by many widows in eighteenth-century France, were reason enough for Cottin to remain unmarried. What was left unsaid, however, may have actually been greater justification in Cottin's mind for steadfastly refusing to remarry. For Sophie Cottin, adamant and publicly avowed disciple of Rousseau, was barren. More importantly, she knew the reason for her sterility, as the evidence we will examine in the following chapter shows. In late-eighteenth-century France, how could a woman who knew she was reproductively "defective" allow herself to be considered by suitors as a legitimate candidate for marriage? This was the crux of Cottin's dilemma, and the novel she began during the summer of 1797, also treated in the next chapter, gives many important insights into the problem.

2
Infertility and Plenitude in *Claire d'Albe*

Il y a des choses que l'on sent si vivement, qu'on voudrait avoir pour en parler d'autres mots que les mots ordinaires.
[There are things one feels so deeply that, to talk about them, one would like to have other than ordinary words.]
—Sophie Cottin

SOPHIE COTTIN WAS CHILDLESS AS A CONSEQUENCE OF PERSISTENT amenorrhea from which she suffered almost all of her mature life. The causes of amenorrhea are multiple and complex.[1] We do not know the causes of Cottin's condition, but she claimed to have suffered from it continually from the time of her marriage on. To discover the facts about her condition as she herself described them, we must skip forward several years to an important letter she wrote in 1805.[2] In his biography of Cottin, Sykes published excerpts from this letter and acknowledged that it dealt with her childlessness but stopped short of offering any explanation for her infertility, though Cottin herself had addressed the problem directly in the letter. We can perhaps attribute this lacuna to Sykes's own sense of propriety. The rules may have been different, however, in 1830, when Henri de Latouche published several letters from Cottin's correspondence, one of which was the unedited version of this letter. It is the best evidence we have of Cottin's view of herself as a "defective" female and a key to understanding the forces at work in her textual production that previous readings, including Sykes's, have failed to take into account.

The letter she wrote in 1805 was addressed to Hyacinthe Azaïs, with whom she had fallen in love during her stay at the thermal hot springs of Bagnères-de-Bigorre in the summer of 1804. I shall delay a detailed discussion of their relationship until later in the study; for now, to understand the context of the letter, it is important to know only that upon her return to Paris, Cottin found it necessary to explain her condition. This letter is perhaps the most self-revealing document in her existing correspondence; with it, she broke a self-imposed silence that had lasted for many years:

> Les devoirs, ne disons pas pourtant qu'ils sont très faciles; car j'en ai un à remplir envers vous qui me coûte sensiblement. C'est la seule pensée qui, relative à moi, et m'occupant continuellement, vous est demeurée cachée jusqu'à ce jour. Dans le commencement de nos liaisons, n'osant vous le dire, j'aurais voulu la confier à Mme de R[ivière]. . . . Vers la fin de mon séjour à Bagnères, cette pensée, qui est une crainte désolante, avait disparu. Je l'ai retrouvée ici [à Paris]: et c'est votre dernière lettre qui m'apprend que c'est pour moi un devoir indispensable de vous le dire. Mais comment s'y prendre? Comment entrer dans ces détails dont la modestie a tant à souffrir? . . . Mon ami, détournez-vous, et écoutez-moi.
> Je lis dans votre dernière lettre: 'Sans l'espérance de voir naître une famille, ce serait un devoir pour nous de ne pas nous unir sur cette terre.'—Mon ami, mon tendre ami, je ne l'ai pas, cette espérance. Voilà le motif qui doit m'excuser à vos yeux, d'avoir, si jeune, renoncé au mariage. Dans les premiers moments où je vous parlais de cette résolution, vous n'y étiez pas intéressé encore; vous la blâmates; je vous dis que si vous en connaissiez les motifs, vous me justifieriez. Voilà le principe, voilà la cause de mon silence, chaque fois que vous me parliez de ce bonheur bien plus doux que notre union même. Voilà la raison secrète qui appuyait toutes celles que je vous donnais pour vous regretter. Ah! si j'avais eu l'espoir d'être mère!
> Je l'ai eu un moment; et c'est alors que j'ai osé redemander de l'amour à votre coeur, et que je me suis engagée à vous appartenir. J'ai dû au long séjour de Bagnères, à son air, à ses eaux, à ses bains, un rétablissement dans ma santé, auquel j'avais renoncé depuis longtemps. Dès l'hiver dernier, j'avais retrouvé ces symptômes qui donnent aux femmes l'espérance du plus grand bonheur; et comme mon coeur a palpité de joie dans ces temps-là! Comme il a osé vous aimer! Comme il s'envirait de la pensée de s'unir à vous, et de vous donner tous les biens! Mon Dieu! Mon Dieu! aimer un être qui vous aurait dû l'existence! Ah, mon ami, où aurais-je trouvé assez d'amour pour l'aimer assez? Non, non, je ne suis pas destinée à une pareille félicité. Depuis mon retour ici, j'en ai perdu toute espérance. Cet accident, particulier à ma santé, existait au moment de mon mariage; je lui ai dû le malheur de n'avoir point d'enfants. Il a duré presque continuellement jusqu'à mon voyage à Bagnères. Lorsqu'il cessa, je crus que Dieu même me montrait qu'il m'avait amenée là pour être à vous. Depuis mon retour, il a bien fallu changer de pensée. Je méditais, dans une silencieuse mélancolie, sur ce que je devais faire. Partout dans votre journal, je voyais vos voeux pour une famille; c'était bien

plus une famille qu'une compagne que vous désiriez. Mon coeur se brisait; le devoir me commandait bien de parler; mais j'étais sûre que vous alliez m'aimer beaucoup moins quand j'aurais parlé, et je ne pouvais me décider à rompre le silence. Pour en avoir la force, il fallait que je m'exaltasse jusqu'à préférer le devoir à votre amour. J'ai combattu longtemps, et la victoire n'est pas complètement gagné.

[Let us not say, nevertheless, that duty is easily done, for I have one in regards to you that comes at a high price for me. It is the only thought that, concerning me and constantly on my mind, has remained hidden from you until now. At the beginning of our relationship, not daring to tell you, I wanted to confess it to Mme de R[ivière]. ... By the end of my stay in Bagnères, this thought, this overwhelming fear, had disappeared. It has returned here [in Paris]: and your last letter has made me realize that it is my unavoidable duty to tell you. But how can I do it? How can I talk about those details that break the laws of modesty? ... My friend, avert your eyes, and listen.

I read in your last letter: "Without the hope of having a family, duty dictates that we should not be united on this earth." My friend, my dear friend, I do not have that hope. This is the reason I renounced marriage at such a young age, a reason that should excuse me in your eyes. When I first spoke to you of that decision, it didn't yet affect you directly; you condemned it; I tell you that if you knew the reasons, you would find me justified in making it. This was the reason for and the cause of my silence each time you spoke to me of a happiness much greater than that of our own marriage. This was the secret reason underlying all those I gave you in resisting your entreaties. Ah! if only I had had the hope of being a mother!

I did have it for a moment; and that is when I dared ask once more for love from your heart and promised to become your wife. Thanks to my long stay in Bagnères, to Bagnères's air, water, and mineral baths, my health was restored, something I had given up on long ago. Beginning last winter, those signs that give a woman hope for the greatest happiness returned; and how my heart rejoiced in those days! How it dared to love you! How giddy it was with the thought of being yours and giving you everything! My God! My God! to love a being that would be indebted to you for its very existence! Ah, my friend, where would I have found enough love to love it adequately? No, no, it is not my lot to know such happiness. Since my return here, I have lost all hope of knowing it. This defect, a characteristic of my particular state of health, existed during my marriage; because of it, I have no children. The condition had persisted almost without change until my trip to Bagnères. When it ended, I believed that God himself was showing me that he had led me there to be your wife. Since my return, I have had to change my mind. I have meditated, in silent melancholy, about what I needed to do. In your journal, I read of your desire for a family everywhere; more than a mate, you wanted a family. My heart was breaking; duty was exhorting me to tell all; but I was certain that you would love me much less after I had spoken, and I could not bring myself to speak. To find the strength, I needed to bring myself to the point of preferring duty over love. I have struggled a long time, and the victory is not yet assured.[3]

This single letter informs us on many levels. First, it shows us how difficult it was for Cottin to talk about her condition; in fact, we can assume from what she says here that no man other than Azaïs ever heard it from her directly. For years, then, infertility was the reason she refused all marriage proposals, infertility the buried thing she could not voice. Second, Cottin makes us aware of the intensity of her desire to have children; maternity is, according to her, "the greatest happiness." Knowing that she could not bring that possibility to a marriage, she considered herself an unfit and defective candidate. And she is certain that Azaïs—or any other man of his century, for that matter—would agree with her on this issue. Third, Cottin's comments reflect the common beliefs of her generation about infertility, beliefs that had been by and large formed by religious dogma. Much of what the average eighteenth-century French person believed about human fertility came from the interpretations of sacred texts, preached from pulpits and perpetuated by priestly counsel in confessional booths for centuries.

The biblical narratives reflecting the pronatalism of ancient Hebrew culture greatly influenced the formation of Western attitudes about fertility and infertility. The scriptural text asserts that God controls procreation. As Jean-Louis Flandrin has pointed out:

It is true that western society had known for millennia that procreation is a result of sexual union. However, because people did not know the details, nor even the fundamental organs of the process of generation, and because it had been observed that sexual relations were not always fertile, one could believe that conception depended immediately on the will of God. By their sexual union, the parents provided the raw material for the future child, but it was God himself who decided whether or not to make a child from this seminal material, and who, in any case, introduced the soul at a particular moment in the process of gestation. This could not be doubted by married couples who waited for years for a conception that never occurred; nor by those who, living a normal sexual life, were, to a greater extent than others, overburdened with children. God sent children to whomsoever He wished, and in such numbers as He wished, and the spouses generally did not imagine that it depended on them to increase or diminish their fertility.[4]

Infertility is a persistent theme in Judeo-Christian scripture. The Hebrew God's first commandment to his new creations in the Garden of Eden, Adam and Eve, was to be "fruitful, and multiply, and replenish the earth" (Gen. 1:28), an injunction repeated to Noah after the earth has been wiped clean by the flood: "And you, be ye fruitful, and multiply; bring forth abundantly in the earth, and multiply therein" (Gen. 9:7). Very early on, Hebraic scripture makes it clear that fertility comes as the result of obedience and is the sign of Jehovah's favor. This is first illustrated with the example of Abraham, whose wife, Sarah, is described as "barren" (Gen. 11:30). When very old, Abraham is told by visiting angels that his wife will become pregnant. Sarah's reaction is one of joy and disbelief; her womb has been fruitless all her life, and her husband is nearly a hundred years old. Surely this will be the greatest of miracles: bringing life from what is apparently dead. And yet, Sarah conceives and gives birth to Isaac. Abraham's faith is further tested by Jehovah, who asks him to prepare their only child for sacrifice. When Abraham passes the test, he is rewarded with the greatest gift Jehovah offers his faithful, namely, an infinite posterity: "I will bless thee, and in multiplying I will multiply thy seed as the stars of the heaven, and as the sand which is upon the sea shore; and thy seed shall possess the gates of his enemies; And in thy seed shall all the nations of the earth be blessed, because thou has obeyed my voice" (Gen. 22:17–18).

Because of scriptural inferences that Jehovah rewarded obedient humans with offspring, infertility came to be seen as a sign of punishment in Hebraic culture, a situation that, even when there was no evidence of overt disobedience, created feelings of guilt and shame in the barren woman. The stories of Rachel and Hannah, for instance, illustrate well this dilemma. Rachel, the favorite wife of Isaac, had no children: "And when Rachel saw that she bare Jacob no children, Rachel envied her sister [Leah]; and said unto Jacob, Give me children, or else I die" (Gen. 30:1). Jacob's response to his wife's demand reflected his understanding of the rules of fertility: "And Jacob's anger was kindled against Rachel: and he said, Am I in God's stead, who hath withheld from thee the fruit of the womb?" (Gen. 30:2). Fortunately, God did have compassion on Rachel "and opened her womb" (Gen. 30:22), and

Rachel gave thanks, praising God for having taken away "[her] reproach" (Gen. 30:23).

Hannah's story gives evidence of the kind of open ridicule barren women suffered in her culture: "[T]he Lord had shut up her womb. And her adversary also provoked her sore, for to make her fret, because the Lord had shut up her womb. . . . [W]hen she went up to the house of the Lord, so [her adversary] provoked her; therefore she wept, and did not eat. Then said Elkanah her husband to her, Hannah, why weepest thou? and why eatest thou not? and why is thy heart grieved? am not I better to thee than ten sons?" (1 Sam. 1:5–8). The answer to that question, as far as Hannah is concerned, is a resounding no. Like Rachel's, however, this story has a happy ending. Hannah strikes a bargain with God: if God will "open her womb," she will dedicate the child to God's service; subsequently, she gives birth to a son, names him Samuel, and turns him over to the chief priest in the temple, where he will be trained to serve. Additional children come to Hannah, implying that her sacrifice qualified her for further rewards.

Interestingly, when the biblical text focuses on infertile women, it is to emphasize their success in overcoming sterility. The text is silent about the others who never escaped their "reproach"; to understand their predicament, we have to imagine a Hannah, sorely provoked by her adversary, weeping in the temple, who never ever gets her Samuel. If we can imagine such a scenario, then we can begin to understand the emotional and psychological impact of infertility on women such as Sophie Cottin.

When in her 1805 letter Cottin talks of the restoration of a normal menstrual cycle while living in Bagnères, she reads it as a sign from God that he was preparing her for marriage with Azaïs. In other words, fertility and the divine were inextricably linked in her mind, as they were for most of her contemporaries. However, by suggesting connections between Bagnères's water and the return of normal menstruation, she also points toward her century's popular beliefs about the efficacy of human intervention in the treatment of infertility.

Eighteenth-century scientists were not agreed on the actual process of fertilization. Some believed the male's semen contained all the necessary material for the new being's growth. This theory, originating in Aristotle, had gained renewed momentum with Anton van Leeuwenhoek's discovery of spermatozoa in 1677.[5] However, William Harvey and others held to the "ovist" theory, believing that the female produced eggs containing the essential form, which semen then merely "excited into life." In both camps, however, it was generally believed that orgasm on the part of both partners was necessary for conception. In the female, orgasm caused the womb to open and receive the male's semen; when, therefore, a woman took no pleasure in the sexual act, the womb remained shut, eliminating the possibility of conception. "The womb must be in a state of delight," wrote John Marten in 1708, for pregnancy to occur.

Some medical authorities believed that an imbalance in a wife's bodily "humors" was as equally to blame for female infertility as frigidity. Western medical practice had, since the Greeks, stressed the necessity of maintaining a proper equilibrium to ensure good health. Too much or too little of one vital component in the body's fluids could throw the rest of the system into disorder. Even when the ancient theory of the "four humors"—blood, phlegm, choler (yellow bile), and melancholy (black bile)—had been largely abandoned, medical practitioners continued to stress the concept of "balance." A fever, for instance, diagnosed as a surplus of blood, was treated by bleeding the patient in order to bring the blood level back to normal. Bladder and bowel evacuations were monitored closely for irregularities. Female problems such as vaginal discharges and menstrual disorders fell naturally into this same category of "imbalances": "Practitioners ranging from the learned European professor of physic to the village midwife agreed that these imbalances might easily lead to sterility."

A very useful example of the thinking in this domain is James Walker's *Inquiry into the Causes of Sterility in Both Sexes,* published in Philadelphia in 1797. A candidate for the degree of doctor of medicine at the University of Pennsylvania, Walker attempted in his thesis to summarize the most recent scientific thought coming out of both Europe and America on the suggested treatment of the condition. In his introduction, Walker acknowledges the serious psychological effects of infertility on the sufferer: "The anxiety of mind, which appears to be universally connected with unfruitful marriages, is found to be the cause of as much evil in the world, as any of those diseases to which we are liable."[6] And yet, Walker points out, medical science has neglected to conduct a methodical inquiry into the problem: "We find little mention made of Sterility, either by the ancient or modern Physicians. . . . I have not been able to find, that any of the moderns have treated of it methodically" (7–8). His thesis is meant to fill a very noticeable gap in the scientific discourse of his time and improve the lives of those suffering from infertility, for "upon inquiry it appears, that many causes of Sterility are not without a remedy" (7).

Walker begins with a review of the most current theories of reproduction, summarizing the opinions of both the animalculists—Leeuwenhoek and others—and the ovists, among whom he cites "the venerable Haller" and "the ingenious Spallanzani," a strong indication of Walker's own theoretical preferences (11). He is careful, however, to draw no definitive conclusions about any of the fertilization process: "This secret operation of nature will probably remain a matter of opinion, as no experiment can ever ascertain it in the human subject" (13). Having said this, Walker moves on to explore what he believes the science of medicine can ascertain, that is, the observable physical causes of sterility. He states: "Barrenness is the effect, not the cause of diseases. . . . I shall confine myself to those [diseases] that are more the immediate causes of Barrenness by affecting the uterine system" (14). The first disorders Walker discusses under this rubric are "those which have the effect of interrupting the menstrual discharge," for, as he posits, "It appears to be the monthly flow of the Menses that capacitates the human female to become pregnant, at all seasons of the year; and it has been observed, that pregnancy very generally takes place soon after one of the periods of their occurence [sic]" (14–15). Walker proposes that menstruation may be disrupted by two different "states of the system," which he designates "Suppression and Retention," "suppression" defined as the disappearance of menstruation after having begun normally during puberty and "retention" defined as a condition "when the menstrual flux does not begin to flow at that time of life which [sic] it should make its appearance" (15). "Suppression" he blames on "a preternatural [abnormal] resistance" of the blood vessels, in particular the vessels of the uterus (15). "Retention," on the other hand, is the result of disease, birth defects, or accidents that prevent the reproductive system from developing normally.

Having established the basic causes for sterility, Walker then moves to a discussion of cures, but not without a warning: "We are not . . . to expect cures in all cases, and indeed but few of them comparatively speaking, according to the number which occur" (20). He suggests that for the treatment of "suppression," the physician must "lessen" the resistance of the vessels of the uterus "by blood letting, and other depleting remedies" (20). Continuing, Walker explains: "Our chief remedy, after the tone of the system is lessened, and the plethora [an excess of blood] removed, is the warm bath, or sitting over the steam of water, . . . which acts by relaxing the coats of the arteries whilst the stimulus of the warmth increases their action" (20–21). In the case of retention, where there is "a want of excitement" and the blood pressure is low, then Walker recommends "stimulants and tonics: the exercise of the lower limbs in walking or dancing is highly serviceable" (21). Bleedings may also be helpful in stimulating the uterus, Walker adds, as well as electric shocks to the pelvic region. In those cases where there is "want of excitement" and a normal menstrual flow, Walker recommends remedies promoting strength: "aliment of a nutricious [sic] nature, the martial mineral waters, and the class of bitters," among which he names clove water (21). "Medicines," he concludes, "will be of little service in barrenness that proceeds from local diseases, except when it is produced by local debility, in which case we should always endeavour to remove the exciting causes, and when this is done the strictest attention should be paid to cleanliness" (21–22).

Walker's *Inquiry* gives us a useful insight into the late-eighteenth-century's approach to infertility. A man of science, he is decidedly cautious in his claims, recognizing from the outset the difficulties inherent in a field where so much was perforce based on conjecture and tradition. Walker's intended readership would have been restricted to those of his own profession, other men of science, for whom the role of the supernatural in the healing arts was not a legitimate subject of scientific inquiry. Hence, other than a quotation from Genesis on the frontispiece—the commandment to "multiply and replenish the earth"—there is no mention of divinity's role in fertility matters in the book. Popular treatises on the subject, however, after listing all the possible remedies for infertility, always ended with the reminder that there was no guarantee of success for, in the final analysis, children were a gift from God.[7]

In the eighteenth century, "Women . . . generally bore the onus of a barren marriage," historians Margaret Marsh and Wanda Ronner have pointed out. "Barrenness . . . was clearly a woman's problem, and self-treatment was the usual means employed to alleviate it."[8] Many women had books listing recipes for homemade medicines—gathered from a variety of sources, including midwives—for the treatment of female problems. Physicians like James Walker had to admit that the cures of the "good old women," as he calls the midwives, were often efficacious and served as the starting point for his own scientific inquiry (7). For those women who could afford it, a visit to one of the well-known mineral spas such as Baden-Baden in Germany or Evian in France was a popular remedy. As we have seen, Walker too recommends steam baths and the ingestion of mineral waters as useful practices in treating sterility. Sophie Cottin gave most of the credit for the restoration of her menstrual cycle to the waters of Bagnères-de-Bigorre, a village in the French Pyrenees. It is also evident that Cottin blamed her return to Paris for the loss of what she had briefly regained in Bagnères.

Cottin's 1805 letter gives us a glimpse into the "anxiety" of infertility which, as a physician, James Walker was anxious to alleviate if possible. No psychologist, this eighteenth-century doctor nevertheless observed correctly that sterility's most damaging consequences are psychological. Modern researchers have attempted to articulate the mental processes involved with infertility that Cottin's letter appears to reflect. As Daniluk, Leader, and Taylor explain:

> For a woman, the inability to produce a child may be perceived as an inability to fulfill her biological role. The experience of infertility is often accompanied by a strong tendency toward self-blame. . . . The resultant frustration, anxiety, and stress often experienced by the infertile individual or couple may have adverse impacts on their self-image, self-esteem, psychological well-being, marital relationship, and sexual satisfaction and functioning. . . . Within the context of a strong, pronatalistic socialization, the inability to achieve such a highly valued and highly reinforced life goal may leave an individual or couple questioning their relationship, physical and psychological health, worthiness, value, and sense of sexual identity. . . . [T]he infertility experience . . . may be prolonged over time and may adversely affect all aspects of the infertile individual's intrapersonal and interpersonal life.[9]

Statistics on infertility in eighteenth-century France are not available to us but we can perhaps build a plausible hypothesis based on modern research showing that "up to 15% of couples in developed countries are involuntarily infertile, with a much higher percentage in developing countries."[10] Barbara Menning, who has devoted much of her life as a scholar to the study of infertility, states: "This population represents one of the most neglected and silent minority groups in our country. They are not sick, merely heartsick. They continue to work, to function, to carry out their lives in a state of involuntary childlessness which can pervade every waking moment and make decisions for the future impossible."[11]

From working with infertile people, modern psychologists have constructed a model explaining the psychological stages through which the infertile person passes in dealing with his or her crisis. In obvious ways, the model resembles the stages of feelings associated with the death of a loved one; indeed, the process appears to be the same, for the infertile person is dealing with loss, the loss of a potential person, the unborn. Barbara Menning and others propose that the infertile person goes through six succeeding phases:

1. Surprise: this is the first reaction, as there exists little preparation for infertility. People do not normally think of themselves as infertile.
2. Denial: some experience shock and disbelief, others may already know they are infertile and exhibit denial by denying their desire for children. Denial may also occur with the failure of infertility treatments. "Denial serves a purpose," Menning claims. "It allows the mind and body to adjust at their own rate to an overwhelming situation."[12] Denial can become dangerous, however, if it becomes long-term.
3. Anger: resulting from feelings of a loss of control, it can be aggravated by societal pressure and others' insensitivity to the problem.
4. Isolation: the impulse to isolation stems from the desire to avoid the pressures and probing of family and society. Infertility is a sensitive, personal issue; the discovery of the lack of understanding in others about the seriousness of the loss causes the sufferer to find ways of escaping from more potential pain.
5. Guilt: interestingly, even in modern society, those struggling with infertility have the feeling that they must have done something wrong to deserve the punishment of infertility. They often seek a way to "atone" for certain actions and assuage guilt. Other aspects of life are affected; the patients feel "unworthy and incapable in every sector."[13] "The losses attached to childlessness may include loss of faith, loss of power, loss of dreams of the future and loss of sexual function and intimacy."[14]
6. Grief: this may be preceded by a period of depression, precipitated by the patient's final realization that he or she will never have children. Depression is different from sadness; it

is, as Jane Read explains, a more "sustained response."[15] As Menning points out, "Society has elaborate rituals to comfort the bereaved in death. Infertility is different. . . . Family and friends may never even know. The infertile couple often comes to this point of grief alone."[16] Menning claims that failure or inability to grieve is the most common problem she has encountered in counseling infertile people. She cites as reasons for this failure to grieve the following: there may be no recognized loss, the loss may be seen as "socially unspeakable," there may be uncertainty about the loss, and there may be an absence of a social support system.[17] The grief process, however, must be completed if the patient is to lead a productive life.[18]

These findings can, I believe, help us to understand better the psychological state of a woman like Sophie Cottin. Thanks to the 1805 letter, we know that she came out of her short-lived marriage childless because of a physical condition and not a choice. The principal cause of her rejection of all offers of remarriage, this "defectiveness" appears to have been preoccupying her as she began writing in earnest during the summer of 1797.

As Sykes has pointed out, writing was not new to her: she had written some poetry and a short story previously, but now writing took on a much greater urgency. She admitted that the world of the imagination might not provide the happiness she sought, but it did give her at least a measure of peace she did not find in the real world: "Quand l'imagination travaille, le coeur repose, et dans le calcul, si la nature murmure, la prudence applaudit, et si le bonheur n'y trouve pas son compte, la tranquillité y trouve le sien" ["When the imagination is at work, the heart reposes, and in the end, if nature protests, prudence applauds, and if happiness doesn't find fulfilment in it, peace of mind does"] (*MC*, 314). A letter written after the publication of *Claire d'Albe* gives another perspective on the production of her first novel: "Seule à la campagne, dans les plus beaux, les plus longs jours de l'année, tourmentée par des souvenirs et par le regret de certaines illusions, je m'amusai à mettre sur le papier une histoire dont le fond est tout d'imagination, mais dont certains sentiments ne me furent pas étrangers" ["Alone in the country, on the longest and most beautiful days of the year, tormented by memories and the loss of certain dreams, I amused myself by writing an essentially imaginary story, but which describes certain feelings I have known"] (329).

Her confession about the autobiographical nature of the feelings, the "loss of certain dreams" expressed in the novel, is perhaps reason enough to explain her decision to have the work published anonymously. The manuscript was turned over to her cousin Lemarcis who, acting as her agent, sold it to the Parisian bookseller Maradan; in a note to Julie, Cottin complained about the money Maradan was willing to pay: "Maradan ne voulait donner que 240 frs.; on n'a pu obtenir que 300 frs" ["Maradan only wanted to pay me 240 francs; we could only get 300 out of him"] (*MC*, 399). Maradan's reticence was understandable in light of the fact that he was gambling on a first book by a woman who insisted on remaining anonymous. Cottin was, however, encouraged by Maradan's first impression of the book and his request that Lemarcis encourage the writer to continue: Maradan "a fait le plus grand éloge de l'ouvrage. Il a prié mon cousin d'engager la dame à travailler encore, et que ce n'était pas seulement son avis, mais celui d'un homme de lettres qu'il avait consulté" ["gave the book his highest praise. He asked my cousin to encourage the writer to produce another book, and told him that this was not only his own opinion, but also that of another author he had consulted"] (399). Cottin then vowed: "Si cet ouvrage réussit, je deviendrai plus difficile pour celui que je vais faire" ["If this work succeeds, I will be more forceful about the next one I do"] (399). The statement is obvious proof that Cottin already had another novel in mind and that she expected to continue to make money from her writing. The *Claire d'Albe* manuscript was in the printer's hands by December 1798 but did not appear in bookstores until the following May. It was an immediate success (43).

Claire d'Albe, the story of a young mother of two who succumbs to an illicit passion, experiencing for the first time in her life the *plénitude* she has desperately sought, inscribes Cottin's personal search to create a viable female identity outside the pronatalistic norms of eighteenth-century French culture. To achieve this, Cottin creates a radically different male gaze that valorizes the heroine, Claire, through her virtues and not her reproductive potentiality.

The epistolary novel begins with a letter in which Claire describes her situation to her best friend Elise. In the course of the letter, she discloses that she had been married seven years earlier, at age fifteen, to a man nearly forty years her elder, the result of a deathbed request by her father. She is now twenty-two years old and the mother of two children, Adolphe and Laure. In the third letter of the series—one Cottin transcribed directly into the novel from a letter she herself had written to a friend—we find that Claire is far from happy: "Ô mon Elise! je ne te tromperai pas, et tu m'as devinée: oui, il est des moments . . . où je soupçonne que mon sort n'est pas rempli comme il aurait pu l'être: ce sentiment, qu'on dit être le plus délicieux de tous, et dont le germe était peut-être dans mon coeur, ne s'y développera pas, et y mourra vierge" ["Oh, Elise, I will not fool you and you have surely guessed; yes, there are moments . . . when I suspect that my destiny has not been fulfilled as it should have been; this feeling, that others call the most delicious of all and of which I carry the seed perhaps in my heart, will never grow there and will die there untouched."][19] Locked in a loveless marriage, Claire feels her situation now precludes any hope of finding this passion that would transform her present unfulfilled life into the ideal: "Ah! laisse-moi sous mes ombrages; c'est là qu'en rêvant un mieux idéal, je trouve le bonheur que le ciel m'a refusé" ["Oh, leave me in my darkness; it is there, dreaming about the ideal, that I find the happiness the heavens have refused me"] (1:398).

Little does she suspect the fate that awaits her; her husband's seemingly harmless invitation to a cousin to stay with them begins a chain of cataclysmic events. This cousin, Frédéric, nineteen years old, has been raised far from civilization; in her description of him to Elise, Claire seems to have found in Frédéric a true child of nature: "Le séjour des montagnes a donné autant de souplesse et d'agilité à son corps, que d'originalité à son esprit et de candeur à son caractère. Il ignore jusqu'aux moindres usages. . . . [J]'aime ce caractère neuf qui se montre sans voile et sans détour, cette franchise crue. . . . Je n'ai point encore vu une physionomie plus expressive" ["Life in the mountains has given as much suppleness and agility to his body as originality to his mind and candor to his character. He is ignorant of the most common customs. . . . I love this new personality that manifests itself without guile, this raw candor. . . . I have never seen a more expressive face"] (1:399). She casts him in the role of the newly created Adam, just entering the world: "C'est un caractère neuf, qui n'a point été émoussé encore par le frottement des usages. Aussi présente-t-il toute la piquante originalité de la nature. On y retrouve ces touches larges et vigoureuses dont l'homme dut être formé en sortant des mains de la Divinité; on y pressent ces nobles et grandes passions qui peuvent égarer sans doute, mais qui, seules, élèvent à la gloire et à la vertu" ["His is a pristine character, the newness of which has not yet been lost through habit's routine. And so he displays all the striking originality of nature.

One finds in him the strong, broad touches that divinity must have used in forming the first man; noble and great passions foreshadow themselves in him, passions that can surely lead one into error but that alone can elevate a man to glory and virtue"] (1:401–2). Claire proves prophetic here: this character, unlike other men in his capacity for great passion, has the capability of great sin as well, but Claire feels drawn to him as to a revelation: "Je l'étudie avec cette curiosité qu'on porte à tout ce qui sort des mains de la nature.... La vérité n'est pas au fond du puits, mon Elise, elle est dans le coeur de Frédéric" ["I am studying him with the kind of curiosity one has about things that come directly from nature.... Truth is not at the bottom of a well, Elise, it is in Frédéric's heart"] (1:403).

Through the character of Frédéric, Cottin constructs a nonpatriarchal male gaze, that is, a gaze other than that of the husband, that measures the flesh-and-blood Claire against an avowed ideal. Frédéric, like Adam, is anxious to find his Eve, the woman whose image he, not God, has created mentally, as he tells Claire: "Dans les premiers beaux jours de ma jeunesse, aussitôt que l'idée du bonheur eut fait palpiter mon sein, je me créai l'image d'une femme telle qu'il la fallait à mon coeur. Cette chimère enchanteresse m'accompagnait partout; je n'en trouvais le modèle nulle part" ["During the first beautiful days of my youth, as soon as the idea of happiness was born in my heart, I created the image of a woman I would need for my heart. This dream enchantress went everywhere with me; but I could find her equal nowhere"] (1:407). The mountain man-child's unique religion was the worship of his phantom woman: "C'est dans ces pays sauvages et sublimes que l'imagination s'exalte et allume dans le coeur un feu qui finit par le dévorer; c'est là que je me créai un fantôme auquel je me plaisais à rendre une sorte de culte" ["In those wild, sublime surroundings, the imagination takes flight and lights a fire in the heart that ends by destroying it; it is there I created a phantom woman for myself that I delighted in worshiping"] (1:426–27).

Cottin demonstrates this "natural" male gaze at work in several crucial scenes in the novel. One of the most important of these episodes occurs when Frédéric happens upon Claire as she is attending to her old nurse, who has suffered an attack of apoplexy. Claire, in describing the event to Elise, relates how the scene affected Frédéric: "Pendant que j'en étais occupée, j'ai entendu une exclamation, et, levant la tête, j'ai vu Frédéric.... Frédéric était en extase: il revenait de la promenade, et, voyant du monde devant la chaumière, il y était entré. Depuis un moment il était là; il contemplait, non plus sa cousine, m'a-t-il dit, non plus une femme belle autant qu'aimable, mais un ange!" ["While I was thus occupied, I heard a cry and looking up, I saw Frédéric. . . . He was in ecstasy; he had just returned from a walk and, seeing a crowd outside the hut, he had entered. He had been there for a moment; he told me he was looking at someone who was no longer his cousin nor a woman as wonderful as she was beautiful, but rather an angel!"] (1:407). Claire must confront this new and discomforting gaze at every turn with Frédéric: "Assis près de moi, il me regardait fixement, trop fixement; c'est là son seul défaut, car son regard a une expression qu'il est difficile, . . . j'ai presque dit dangereux de soutenir" ["Seated next to me, he was watching me transfixed, too transfixed; that is his only defect, for his gaze has an expression difficult, . . . I almost said dangerous, to endure"] (1:412). She is painfully aware of being evaluated against the strictest of standards.

Significantly, however, none of these crucial evaluation scenes display Claire in her mothering duties and, even more importantly, when Frédéric openly praises her virtues as a woman, he makes no direct mention of her role as a mother. This is in direct contrast to the husband, M. d'Albe, who, whenever discussing his wife with Frédéric in their man-to-man conversations, never once fails to emphasize Claire's maternal skills. Frédéric, then, the young man born and reared in the mountains and hence ignorant of the cultural norms of the dominating class, ascribes value to Claire based on her abilities to inspire devotion in her mate *outside* the field of maternity.

As a corollary to this, Frédéric steadfastly downplays Claire's physical attributes in favor of her moral virtues. When asked to comment on a portrait recently painted of Claire, he insists: "Non, non, des traits sans vie ne rendront jamais Claire; et là où je ne vois point d'âme, je ne puis la reconnaître" ["No, no, lifeless features will never portray Claire; and where I can see no soul, I cannot recognize her"] (1:418). If outward appearance had mattered most for him, he tells Claire, he would have chosen Adèle—her beautiful but superficial cousin—over her, but his attraction to Claire is based on his love of goodness: "Je veux t'aimer, parce que tu es ce qu'il y a de meilleur au monde" ["I want to love you because you are what is best in the world"] (1:430).

The portrait episode in *Claire d'Albe* appears to be a direct subversion or rewriting of a similar episode in Rousseau's *La nouvelle Héloïse* in which Saint-Preux, like Frédéric, is shown a portrait of the beloved. Saint-Preux, like Frédéric, rejects the portrait as being unfaithful to the original—in this case, Julie—but then turns the moment to erotic advantage by carefully cataloguing each precise physical detail of Julie's anatomy—so well known to him, the admirer—that had been left out of the artist's rendering. Nowhere in Rousseau's text is the male gaze more blatantly obvious than in the portrait episode. Cottin's Frédéric, in sharp contrast, does not share this male myopia with Saint-Preux; when he looks at Claire, his gaze refuses to stop at surface details but penetrates to revel in the sight of her soul's beauty: "Peu à peu je découvris en vous . . . une âme plus élevée, plus tendre et plus délicate; je vous vis alternativement douce, sublime, touchante, irrésistible; tout ce qu'il y a de beau et de grand vous est si naturel, qu'il faut vous voir de près pour vous apprécier" ["Little by little, I discover in you . . . a more elevated, a more tender and delicate soul; I see you alternately sweet, sublime, touching, irresistible; everything that is beautiful and grand is so natural for you that one has to see you up close to appreciate you"] (1:427). And for Frédéric, seeing Claire "up close" means watching her benevolence at work in her interactions with others.

This is but the first of Cottin's major intertextual confrontations in *Claire d'Albe* with Rousseau's *Héloïse*. Another and perhaps more significant one is her subversion of an ideological position central to Rousseau's text, that is, the primacy of Father's law and its concomitant notions of "duty," which translate into the subjugation and control of female passion. Cottin makes the parallels too obvious to ignore: Claire, like Rousseau's Julie, has married her father's friend. In M. d'Albe's case, he resembles Claire's father so much in both age and demeanor as to be almost his double. To further strengthen the image, Frédéric is considered the adopted son of M. d'Albe, and he literally refers to him as his father. Claire's horror at the thought of an illicit passion for Frédéric stems in large part from her Phèdre-like realization that she is guilty of an incestuous attraction: "Quoi! sous les yeux du plus respectable des hommes, mon époux, parjure à mes serments, j'aimerais le fils de son adoption? . . . Ô honte! chaque mot que je trace est un crime, et j'en détourne la vue en frémissant" ["What, right in front of the most respectable of men, my spouse, unfaithful to my vows, I would love his adopted son? . . . Oh, shame! each word I write is a crime, and trembling I turn my eyes away"] (1:432).

Thus the crime against the husband becomes, for the two

young people, also a crime against Father. Claire exclaims to Frédéric: "Malheureux! me suis-je écriée, oublies-tu que ton bienfaiteur, que ton père est l'époux de celle que tu oses aimer?" ["Unfortunate soul, I cried out, do you forget that your benefactor, your father, is the spouse of the woman you dare to love?"] (1:422). When Claire at last confesses to Frédéric, "Oui, je t'aime avec ardeur, avec violence" ["Yes, I love you passionately, violently"] (1:437), she knows full well the depth of her treason but nevertheless chooses to act to fulfill her own ardent desire. Describing the first forbidden kiss, she writes: "A ce moment, tout a disparu, devoirs, époux, honneur; Frédéric était l'univers, et l'amour, le délicieux amour, mon unique pensée" ["At that moment, everything disappeared: duty, spouse, honor: Frédéric was the universe, and love, delightful love, my only thought"] (1:437).

The plot takes an interesting turn at this juncture in the novel. The fear of sinning against Father is strong enough to make Claire ask Frédéric to leave her home and live with Elise, which he does grudgingly. Elise and M. d'Albe, hoping to kill Claire's attraction to Frédéric, inform her that Frédéric has renewed his relationship with Adèle, Claire's cousin. Claire then refuses to correspond with Frédéric; he takes her silence to mean that she no longer loves him. Both begin to weaken physically. When Frédéric finally uncovers the conspiracy, he races to find Claire to explain all and discovers her near death on the steps of her father's tomb. In explaining what has happened, they realize the extent of the husband/father's deception: "[O]n nous faisait mourir victimes l'un de l'autre, on voulait que nous enfonçassions mutuellement le poignard dans nos coeurs" ["[T]hey were making us kill one another; they wanted us to sink the dagger into one another's heart"] (1:467).

Frédéric then offers Claire a completely different paradigm for living, antithetical to Father's cultural law, passionately declaring: "Crois-moi, Claire, amitié, foi, honneur, tout est faux dans le monde; il n'y a de vrai que l'amour, il n'y a de réel que ce sentiment puissant et indestructible qui m'attache à ton être, et qui, dans ce moment même, te domine ainsi que moi: ne le combats plus, ô mon âme! livre-toi à ton amant; partage ses transports, et, sur les bornes de la vie où nous touchons l'un et l'autre, goûtons, avant de la quitter, cette félicité suprême qui nous attend dans l'éternité" ["Believe me, Claire, friendship, faith, honor, everything is false in the world; the only true thing is love, the only real thing is this powerful indestructible feeling that binds me to you and that, at this very moment, is overpowering you as well as me. Do not fight it any longer, my love; yield to your lover, share his rapture, and on the brink of death, let us experience that supreme joy that awaits us in eternity"] (1:467).

The Adamic male thus sanctions Claire's pursuit of plenitude as a woman in her own right. In direct contrast to Rousseau's Julie, who submits to Father's notions of female maternal "devoir," obediently repressing the love for Saint-Preux she knows to be her only true happiness, Cottin's heroine chooses Frédéric over Father. Instead of dying together as human sacrifices before the urn of the dead Father, they consummate their love on the very steps of his tomb in the ultimate act of rebellion against his will. Significantly, Cottin turns the description of this moment over to Elise who, as a corroborating witness to ecstasy, summarizes rather matter of factly: "Elle l'a goûté dans toute sa plénitude cet éclair de délice qu'il n'appartient qu'à l'amour de sentir; elle l'a connue cette jouissance délicieuse et unique, rare et divine comme le sentiment qui l'a créée: son âme, confondue dans celle de son amant, nage dans un torrent de volupté" ["She tasted in all its fullness that ecstasy that only love can give; she knew that delicious and unique pleasure, rare and heavenly like the feeling that creates it; her soul, lost in that of her lover, swam in a flood of sensual delight"] (1:467). The change of narrative voice used here by Cottin moves us outside of Claire herself to reinforce the textual truth of her experience; the witness voice thus validates the achievement of *plénitude* so ardently desired.

In the end, however, Father is still strong enough to demand that Frédéric be sacrificed. As Claire lies dying, she confesses her sin to her husband and tells him, "ce fut alors que, cessant d'être moi-même, je cessai d'exister pour vous" ["it was then that ceasing to be myself, I ceased to exist for you"] (1:471). Claire then passes out from under Father's domination forever, whispering the forbidden name of Frédéric with her last breath.

Significantly, Elise records the culmination of the tale so that it may be read to Claire's daughter after her mother's death, ostensibly to demonstrate the consequences of illicit passion. But the fervor of the telling betrays the fascination with and attraction of the great moment of *plénitude*. No other passage in the narrative is told with such persuasive energy. The double-edged tale speaks both for and against heterodoxy, its didactic intention subverted by the impassioned voice of Elise. So what does mother *really* want daughter to learn through the telling?

Some contemporary women readers detected immediately the double-barreled message of Cottin's novel. Madame de Genlis, herself a well-established novelist, dismissed it as "un mauvais ouvrage, sans intérêt, sans imagination, sans vraisemblance et d'une immoralité révoltante. . . . [I]l est le premier [roman] où l'on ait représenté l'amour délirant, furieux et féroce, et une héroïne 'vertueuse, religieuse, angélique' et se livrant sans mesure et sans pudeur à tous les emportemens [sic] d'un amour effréné et criminel" ["a bad book, without real interest, without imagination, without verisimilitude and revoltingly immoral. . . . [I]t is the first [novel] in which someone has described delirious love, furious and ferocious love, and a 'virtuous, religious and angelic' heroine, without restraint or virtue, letting herself enjoy all the passions of an unbridled and illicit love"].[20] Genlis, in her commentary on Cottin, gave a synopsis of the novel for her readers but stopped short of quoting Elise's tantalizing description of the love scene, which Genlis found scandalous: "Il faut s'arrêter. . . . Non-seulement une femme, mais un homme qui aurait quelque respect pour le public, n'oserait transcrire la page infâme et dégoûtante qui suit, . . . dont l'extravagance et l'impiété font toute l'énergie" ["I must stop here. . . . Any man, let alone any woman, who respects the reading public would refuse to transcribe the infamous and disgusting page that follows, . . . whose excessive and sacrilegious nature gives it all its power"] (354–55). After quoting Claire's deathbed request, "Que [ma fille] sache que ce qui m'a perdue est d'avoir coloré le vice du charme de la vertu" ["Let [my daughter] know that painting vice with virtue's charms destroyed me"], Genlis asks perspicaciously: "A quoi servent quelques lignes raisonnables, lorsque, dans le cours de l'ouvrage, on n'a cherché qu'à 'colorer le vice du charme de la vertu'?" ["What purpose do these few reasonable lines serve, when, throughout the entire work, the author has tried to 'paint vice with virtue's charms'?"] (356). And, Genlis continues, what other supposedly edifying images are placed before the reader of this "coupable et misérable production?" ["wicked and miserable work?"] (356). The list is damning, she says: sinners discussing virtue, wise men admiring adulterous lovers, illicit passions made into a religion, and finally suicide promoted as an honorable act (357).

For Genlis, the greatest of Claire's—and Cottin's—transgressions was her infidelity to the principles of motherhood. Claire leads her daughter toward crime through the snarelike narrative she insists be told. In addition, Claire's devotion to her lover is antithetical to maternal instinct. To illustrate, Genlis cites Claire's passionate declaration to Frédéric—"c'est par toi seul que j'existe, et pour toi seul que je respire" ["I exist only because of you and for you only do I live"]—to which she attaches this acidic footnote: "Cette sensible Claire a des enfans [*sic*]" ["This sensitive Claire has children"] (350). The blasphemy against motherhood is all too apparent for Genlis and unforgivable coming from a woman writer.

And so the first *jaillissement* of Cottin's heart, the anonymous *Claire*, was read by some as revolutionary and morally subversive. Cottin's heroine seeking fulfillment outside the ascribed norms of fertility and maternity was indeed culturally—and perhaps politically—anarchical in her attempt to escape the control of the father-dominated culture in which she lived. Her rebellion even in death, dying with her lover's name on her lips, provides us with a striking example of a woman rewriting the "old plot," to extend Nancy Miller's analysis of other women novelists, as "a critique of the available cultural solutions."[21] Sophie Cottin incorporated into this text her struggle as a barren woman, living in a culture that refused to grant her value without motherhood. Though she continued to subscribe publicly to the role expected of her sex, *Claire d'Albe* bears the traces of the battle being fought within herself.

3
Back in Step with Jean-Jacques: *Malvina*

MADAME DE GENLIS BLAMED THE APPEARANCE OF *CLAIRE D'ALBE* ON the time period from which it sprang, considering the novel a product fit for consumption only by revolutionaries and their breed. There is no question that Sophie Cottin had had personal experience with the Revolution. Her name, placed on the list of *émigrés* in 1794 as a result of the trips she had made to England and Spain with her husband in 1792, was provisionally removed in April 1796, but with the passage of the law of 5 September 1797 that demanded that all *émigrés* on the list leave France within two weeks, Cottin was once again under pressure. She requested a passport from the ministry of police; her intention, as she indicated to the police, was to leave France on 14 September 1797. We know for certain, however, that she never left Paris.

In January 1798, notification that the police were looking for her as well as a relative of her deceased husband, Madame de Guéroult-Fréville, sent the two into hiding. For six weeks, friends and relatives in Paris and the surrounding area took turns hiding them; letters and packets for them were left at a drop-off point, addressed to "les citoyennes Corbet" (*MC*, 35). Cottin kept up a regular correspondence with Julie, to whom she reaffirmed her enduring attachment: "C'est, dans ce chaos, le seul sentiment qui m'identifie avec tous les points de ma vie. C'est le fil bienfaisant qui m'a été donné pour me conduire et sortir du labyrinthe du monde, c'est lui seul qui me fait sentir que je suis encore moi, car nul autre que le coeur de Sophie ne peut t'aimer comme je t'aime" ["In this chaos, it is the only feeling that connects me with all the points of my life. It is the salutary thread given to me to guide me and bring me out of the labyrinth of the world, it alone makes me feel that I am still myself, for no other heart but the heart of Sophie can love you as I do"] (319).

Cottin asked Julie to intervene on her behalf with the government; she was sure that it would not take much to have her name removed from the list, because she was a woman "qui ne s'est jamais mêlée d'aucune affaire" ["who never got mixed up in any political affairs"] and whose small fortune "la laisse dans l'obscurité qu'elle aime" ["leaves her in the anonymity she loves"] (*MC*, 319). Julie presented the authorities with a petition on 1 March 1798. Cottin evidently felt so sure that her request would be favorably received that she moved back to her home on the chaussée d'Antin by the end of the month. In actuality, her name was not removed until eight months later, on 13 November (35). To be taken off the list, one had to convince the authorities that one had lived in France without interruption since 1 January 1792. It is obvious from this fact that Cottin, Julie, and all concerned had fabricated a persuasive but certainly false representation of Cottin's activities over the preceding five years.

Perhaps because of the police scare, or more likely because of her disenchantment with city life, Cottin moved back to Champlan with Julie and the girls sometime in March or April 1798. In November 1799, she wrote to her sister-in-law, Madame Jauge, who was still in exile in England:

> Voici le cinquième hiver que nous comptons passer encore à la campagne; je crois que la santé de Julie s'en trouvera bien, et notre goût nous y porte davantage chaque jour. La paix et la solitude sont devenues les premiers besoins de ma vie, et les plus chers éléments de mon bonheur. Je vois presque avec effroi l'instant où l'éducation des filles de mon amie nous obligera à faire un plus long séjour à Paris, et si je n'avais l'idée d'y vivre toujours au sein d'une famille à laquelle je suis attachée par les liens les plus étroits et les plus durables, je ne sais si ma cousine pourrait obtenir de moi de quitter mon obscure et paisible retraite.

> [This is the fifth winter that we expect to spend here in the country; I believe Julie's health will be the better for it, and every day we feel more and more comfortable here. Peace and solitude have become the first priorities in my life, and the most vital elements of my happiness. I await almost with dread the moment when the education of my friend's daughters will require us to spend more time in Paris, and if I did not have the prospect of living there surrounded by a family to whom I am attached by the closest and strongest of ties, I don't know if my cousin could get me to leave my obscure and peaceful hideaway.] (*MC*, 326–27)

Newly reinstalled in Champlan, Cottin began writing a second novel, which would turn out almost four times as long as *Claire d'Albe*. She knew, in her heart, however, that writing novels as an agreeable pastime for a woman would certainly not conform to Rousseau's model of female domesticity. There would thus have to be a very compelling, convincing reason for continuing in such a direction. Though her sister-in-law, Marguerite—still in exile in Bath—was the actual reader of the very long letter in which Cottin defended her decision to write a second novel, it is also easy to see, by her rhetorical stance and the arguments she fields, that Rousseau himself is her implied interlocutor. And her answer to him—and any other male detractors, for that matter—is that she is an exception. Relieved of the primordial Rousseauian female roles of wife and mother—the first by her widowhood and the second by her infertility—Cottin could justify her choice:

> Ne croyez pas pourtant, ma soeur, que je sois partisane des femmes auteurs, tant s'en faut. . . . Il me semble que la nature ne donna un coeur si tendre aux femmes, qu'afin de leur faire attacher tout leur bonheur dans les seuls devoirs d'épouse et de mère, et ne les priva de toute espèce de génie que pour ôter à leur vanité le vain désir d'être plus qu'elles ne doivent; que s'il est permis à quelques-unes d'exercer leur plume, ce ne peut être que par exception, et lorsque leur situation les dégage de ces devoirs, qui sont comme la vie du reste de leur sexe.

> [Do not think, however, dear sister, that I am a supporter of women authors, heaven forbid. . . . It seems to me that nature gave women such a tender heart only so as to make them find all their happiness in their sole duties as a wife and mother, and deprived them of any sort of genius only in order to eliminate from their vanity the fruitless desire to be more than they ought to be; if some [women] are permitted to use a quill, it can only be as an exception and when their situation frees them from those duties that are as life itself for the rest of their sex.] (*MC*, 330)

Cottin was sure of the types of things women authors should and should not write about: "Et alors même, je veux qu'elles sentent assez leur insuffisance pour ne traiter que des choses qui demandent de la grâce, de l'abandon et du sentiment" ["And even then, I want them to feel inadequate enough to write only about those things that require grace, ease, and emotion"] (*MC*, 330). Cottin then cautioned her sister-in-law: "Je voudrais bien pourtant, ma bonne amie, que vous ne me lisiez jamais: je crains votre censure, elle me serait plus pénible que celle de tout autre, car un des plus vifs chagrins que je pourrais éprouver, serait de perdre dans votre opinion" ["Nevertheless, my dear friend, I would prefer that you never read my novels: I fear your disapproval, which for me would be more painful coming from you than from anyone else, for losing your respect would cause me the deepest sorrow"] (330). Cottin appears especially worried here that Marguerite will read *Claire d'Albe*, which her sister-in-law would surely find a troubling text, difficult to reconcile with Sophie Cottin's life.

Cottin admitted to Marguerite that her second novel was intended to be a "correction" of *Claire:*

> L'entière certitude que j'avais, en écrivant [*Claire d'Albe*], que jamais on n'en soupçonnerait l'auteur, m'y avait fait répandre des couleurs un peu voluptueuses, des passions un peu vives. Aussi une des plus vives contrariétés que j'aie éprouvées en ma vie, est d'avoir été reconnue lorsque je m'y attendais si peu, et qu'il me semblait avoir pris toutes les précautions nécessaires pour éviter ce chagrin.—Mais alors, me direz-vous, pourquoi publiez-vous un autre roman?—D'abord parce que celui-ci [*Malvina*] est un peu *la correction de l'autre*, que le motif qui m'engage à le livrer à l'impression pallie à mes yeux presque tous les inconvénients, que d'ailleurs ces inconvénients étaient presque tous pour le premier [*Claire*], et puisque j'ai souffert tout ce que j'en pouvais souffrir, je ne vois pas pourquoi je me priverais désormais de l'occupation la plus amusante que j'aie trouvée encore.

> [The absolute certainty that I had, in writing [*Claire d'Albe*], that no one would ever guess the identity of the author, allowed me to include passages a little too passionate. Thus one of the greatest embarrassments of my life was to be recognized when I least expected it, and when it seemed to me that I had taken all the necessary precautions to avoid this difficulty. "Why then," you will ask, "are you writing another novel?" First, because [*Malvina*] is somewhat *a correction of the other*, because, in my opinion, the motivation that drives me to publish it causes all the negative aspects to pale in comparison, because besides, all those negative aspects were tied to the first [*Claire*], and since I have already suffered all I could have suffered on its account, I do not see why for the rest of my life I should deprive myself of the most enjoyable pastime I have yet discovered.] (*MC*, 330, emphasis added)

Realizing how defensive she had been, she apologized: "Mais en voilà bien assez sur ce sujet. Je m'y suis un peu étendue, parce que, pour m'excuser à vos yeux, je sentais que j'avais besoin de toutes les circonstances qui peuvent me justifier d'avoir [*sic*] entré dans cette carrière" ["But enough on this topic. I have belabored the point because, in order to excuse myself in your eyes, I felt I needed all the evidence that could justify my decision to begin this career] (330).

An analysis of *Malvina*'s principal characters, its events and eventual outcome reveals the efforts Cottin took to bring her writing back into step with Rousseau's social philosophy. The revelation of her authorship of *Claire*, as Cottin admitted to Marguerite, had forced her to confront once more the Rousseauian model of female domesticity she had publicly espoused. Malvina, the chaste adoptive mother of a dead friend's daughter who refuses to yield to an empassioned lover's advances because it would separate her from the child she has sworn to protect and raise, thus replaces the rebellious wife-mother Claire.

The novel opens with Malvina crying at the tomb of her best friend, Clara. The narrator informs us that Malvina had been widowed at twenty-one—having never loved her husband—and that she had left France and her fortune to live with Clara, who was married to an English lord. In the house of her friend, she had experienced three years of happiness, "les seuls instants heureux de sa vie" ["the only happy moments of her life"], we are told (2:3). Before dying, Clara had persuaded her husband to promise to let Malvina take complete charge of their five-year-old daughter and her education.

After Clara's death, Lord Sheridan appears all too happy to get rid of Malvina and the child. Malvina receives permission from a relative of her mother, Mistress Birton, to come to Scotland to live. Before leaving, she visits the tomb of Clara once more:

> Elle fut redire à l'ombre de milady Sheridan le serment qu'elle avait prononcé sur son lit de mort; elle fut s'engager une seconde fois à consacrer sa vie entière à l'éducation de Fanny, à ne jamais partager son temps et son affection entre elle et un autre objet. Elle fut promettre enfin de renoncer pour jamais à l'amour; serment téméraire sans doute, que l'exaltation de l'amitié dicta avec ferveur, qu'une mère mourante reçut avec transport, et que la certitude d'avoir adouci par lui les derniers moments de son amie fit renouveler à Malvina avec un pieux enthousiasme.

[She went to repeat to [Clara's] shade the vow she had made at her death; she went to commit herself a second time to consecrate her entire life to Fanny's education, to never divide her time and her affection between [Fanny] and something else. Finally, she went to promise never to love—surely a brave resolve, generated in the fervor of friendship and received with joy by a dying mother, a vow that Malvina, certain of having made her friend's final moments more bearable because of it, now renewed with religious conviction.] (2:3)

Malvina, recognizing the unique nature of this promise, declares: "moi seule, je n'aimerai plus" ["I alone will love no more"] (2:4).

Her relative Mistress Birton serves as a perfect foil to Malvina's model of self-sacrifice and maternal devotion. Mistress Birton lives in a Gothic castle in a mountainous region of Scotland. The castle has a hothouse with exotic plants; the main bedroom, described as an "asile de la volupté" ["a sanctuary of pleasure"] resembles a garden complete with the scent of flowers piped in (2:11). The text points out that the bedroom is a shocking contrast to the charitable hospital that could have been built with the same money, but Birton says she has already done many charitable things, having financed, among other things, a hospital, a school, and a forge. Commenting on Mistress Birton's professed charity, the resident spiritual advisor, M. Prior, notes: "L'amour-propre a été, je le crains bien, le seul et unique mobile de cette action" ["Vanity has been, I fear, the one and only motivation for this behavior"] (2:31). Evidently, Mistress Birton wants to become famous for her charitable work in the mountains around her "palais de fée" ["fairy castle"] (2:31).

When Malvina meets Sir Edmond Seymour, the nephew of Mistress Birton, she falls immediately in love with him. Malvina soon learns, however, that Mistress Birton will assure Edmond his fortune only if he marries Lady Sumerhill, the Sumerhills being one of Scotland's oldest families and one of the most favored in London. If the marriage takes place as planned, Edmond will be guaranteed a seat in Parliament and enough land to make his aunt a "lady." Edmond, however, is a notorious womanizer, openly opposed to the idea of marriage. The text points out, "L'amour, le véritable amour lui fut et lui sera toujours inconnu: ce n'est pas dans un coeur profané par la débauche qu'il allumera jamais ses feux" ["Love, true love was and would ever be unknown to him: love will never light its fire in a heart desecrated by debauchery"] (2:36). Nevertheless, Edmond recognizes that Malvina holds the power to rejuvenate a sinner like himself, and Malvina begins to see how she can be the intermediary through which he can be reborn: "Sir Edmond, dépouillé de ses anciens goûts, renonçant pour jamais aux pernicieuses erreurs qui l'avaient égaré, recommençait pour elle une existence dont il lui devrait tout le bonheur" ["Sir Edmond, stripped of his former appetites, renouncing forever the evil ways that had caused him to stray, was, for her sake, beginning a new life, the happiness of which he would owe to her"] (2:119–20). Edmond writes to his friend: "je ne m'approche du lieu où elle est qu'avec le frémissement religieux qu'on éprouve en entrant dans un temple: je dépose à son aspect tout sentiment, toute pensée qui ne seraient pas dignes d'elle, son souffle divin épure tout ce qui l'approche, et, tant que je suis sous l'ombre de ses regards, je me sens à l'abri du démon" ["I never approach the place where she is without experiencing the religious emotion one feels upon entering a church: seeing her, I leave behind every feeling, every thought unworthy of her, her divine breath purifies everything that comes near her, and, as long as I am beneath her gaze, I feel protected from the devil"] (2:58–59). He closes his letter to his friend: "Charles, lorsque je contemple cette aimable innocence, cette douce fraîcheur, cette beauté sans tache, image de la nature au premier printemps du monde, sans doute je ne me crois pas digne de la posséder; mais en même temps je jure du fond de mon âme que nul autre que moi ne la possédera jamais" ["Charles, when I look upon this wonderful innocence, this charming freshness, this beauty without blemish, the very image of nature in the world's first springtime, surely I do not feel myself worthy to possess it; but at the same time I swear deep down in my soul that no one other than myself will ever possess it"] (2:60).

Malvina's promise to her dying friend, however, precludes, in her own mind at least, any possibility of ever accepting Edmond's affection. While dreaming about Edmond, she is brought up short by the memory of Clara's last words: "il m'en souvient de cet instant affreux où, la remettant dans mes bras, tu me dis: Deviens sa mère, Malvina; qu'elle vive toujours près de toi: étrangère à tout autre pouvoir, je t'impose des devoirs rigoureux, je le sais, mais ce n'est pas à toi que je demanderais un sacrifice ordinaire" ["I remember that terrible moment when, placing her in my arms, you said to me: Become her mother, Malvina; may she always live near you: free as you are of all other ties, I know I am imposing a heavy responsibility on you, but I would not ask any commonplace sacrifice of a woman like you"] (2:120). In a later passage, Malvina and Edmond discuss the virtues of her deceased friend, and Malvina reveals how her promise, like the fall from grace itself, has cast her into a desolate world, shutting her off perpetually from Edenic bliss:

> Hélas! plus je connais le monde, plus je ressens toute l'étendue de la perte que j'ai faite. Il fut un coeur tendre et vrai, sir Edmond, un seul,

sans doute, que le mensonge ne souilla jamais; le ciel l'offrit de bonne heure à mes regards, j'appris à l'aimer en commençant à vivre. Dans l'âme de Clara régnait la franchise, la pureté; on eût dit que toutes les vertus s'y étaient réfugiées; et en la perdant, comme l'Eve de Milton chassée de l'Eden, je suis descendue sur une terre malheureuse et désenchantée par de pénibles comparaisons. —Ah! reprit sir Edmond avec émotion, ignorez-vous donc qu'il est un autre Eden que celui de l'amitié, mille fois plus doux, plus enchanteur, autant au-dessus du sien que le bonheur l'est du repos? —Quand je le croirais, répliqua-t-elle, en s'efforçant de sourire, je n'en serais pas plus heureuse, puisque j'ai juré de n'y jamais entrer.

[Alas! the more I know the world, the more I understand the extent of my loss. There was once upon a time a true and tender heart, Sir Edmond, one alone, surely, that falsehood never sullied; the heavens offered it to me in my early years, I learned to love it as I began my life. Honesty and purity reigned in Clara's soul; you could say that all the virtues lived there; and in losing her, like Milton's Eve thrown out of Eden, I have fallen into an unhappy and disenchanted world by comparison.

"Ah!" answered Sir Edmond with emotion, "are you not aware that there is another Eden, different from that of friendship, a thousand times sweeter, more enchanting, as superior to it as happiness is to repose?"

"Even if I believed that," she replied, trying to smile, "I wouldn't be any happier, because I have sworn never to enter there."] (2:69–70)

Her duty as mother to Fanny thus shuts Malvina off from Edmond. One might argue that Malvina is not a mother in the strictest sense of the term, but the narrator makes it very clear in another episode—one in which Fanny is lost and later found—that Cottin's heroine, without actually being the natural mother of the child, nevertheless has the inborn capability of behaving in all ways like a true mother. Malvina, then, comes very close to being that "exception" that Cottin felt herself to be. It is only when the adopted daughter herself, Fanny, insists that Malvina marry that Malvina feels she has been freed of her vow and gives her hand to Edmond.

But a happy ending is not to be. The natural father of Fanny, Lord Sheridan, upon learning of Malvina's plan to marry, declares that he will turn Fanny over to Mistress Birton to raise if Malvina goes through with her plan. Malvina is thus forced once more to decide between the child and the lover, and she tells Edmond that there will be no marriage. Edmond claims love should take precedence over reason and duty, even morality, but Malvina is not so sure:

> —Et la conscience, Edmond, est-il un bonheur que ses reproches n'empoisonneraient pas?
> —Malvina, quand l'amour n'est pas une flamme qui échauffe, mais un feu qui brûle, qui consume, qui dévore, il étouffe tout, tout, jusqu'à la conscience.
> ["And our conscience, Edmond, is there any happiness that its reproaches would not poison?"
> "Malvina, when love is not merely a flame but rather a raging fire that consumes and devours, it smothers everything, everything, even our conscience."] (2:213)

The contrast between this exchange and that between Frédéric and Claire on the steps of the father's tomb in *Claire d'Albe* is striking; we will remember that Claire succumbs to Frédéric's persuasive rhetoric about love without conscience. Here, in the novelistic antidote to *Claire* that *Malvina* represents, Malvina stands firm on her resolve to remain chaste. Malvina finally shoves Edmond away and tells him to leave. She wants to see him only after he meets with Lord Sheridan in an attempt to get in his good graces and make him relent in his vow. Edmond insists they get married secretly first, however; against her better judgment, Malvina is persuaded to go along with the plan.

Edmond leaves shortly after their marriage to find Lord Sheridan. While he is away, Mistress Birton, by means of a fake letter, leads Malvina to believe that her new husband has been unfaithful to her. When Malvina reads the letter, she is immediately overcome not with anger but rather with overwhelming guilt, for she knows in her heart that she is being punished for having broken her promise to her friend: "Le coup est porté, et mon sort est rempli; *je l'ai bien mérité*" ["The blow has struck home and my fate is decided; *I deserved it only too well*"] (2:237). Mistress Birton makes Malvina choose between dissolving her marriage or keeping Fanny. Malvina resists; there follows a terrible scene describing the separation of Fanny and Malvina:

> —Ils m'ont enlevé mon enfant! s'écria Malvina éperdue et se précipitant hors de la chambre. —Maman! maman! appelait l'enfant en se débattant entre les bras de ceux qui l'emmenaient, est-ce que tu ne viens pas avec moi? —Non, je ne te quitterai pas, lui cria Malvina en se jetant sous les roues de la voiture; et ils m'écraseront, les barbares, avant de t'enlever à ta mère.

["They have stolen my child!" Malvina cried out desperately, running from the room.

"Mama! Mama!" called the child, struggling in the arms of those taking her away, "aren't you coming with me?"

"No, I will never leave you," Malvina cried, throwing herself under the wheels of the carriage, "and they will have to crush me, the brutes, before they take you away from your mother."] (2:253)

The stress from this dilemma takes its toll on Malvina and she becomes delirious, imagining she sees Clara bringing her before the bar of justice of God and crying: "Qu'as-tu fait de mon enfant? qu'as-tu fait de mon enfant?" ["What have you done with my child? What have you done with my child?"] (2:256). Edmond leaves to find Fanny and bring her back; he realizes correctly that the loss of Fanny, not his alleged infidelity, has been the cause of Malvina's insanity: "j'ose attendre beaucoup de la présence de cette enfant; il me semble que l'idée de l'avoir perdue est ce qui trouble le plus Malvina" ["I expect great results from the child's presence; it appears to me that the thought of losing her is what agitates Malvina the most"] (2:256). But Malvina is dying and she gives instructions to her adopted daughter's new caretaker: "Et vous, Mistress Clare, *apprenez surtout à Fanny à ne jamais sacrifier le devoir à l'amour*" ["And you, mistress Clare, *teach Fanny especially never to sacrifice duty for love*"] (2:267; emphasis added). And the novel closes with this scene. In Cottin's first novel, Claire, a mother of two children, dies because she is not allowed to love freely; in her second novel, the heroine Malvina dies because she breaks a vow to be a mother above all else. With *Malvina*, then, Cottin appears to have reaffirmed her allegiance to Rousseau, at least momentarily.

In January 1799, Cottin wrote to Julie to say that she had given her *Malvina* manuscript to André Cottin, her brother-in-law, to read and critique. Almost a year later, in December 1799, Cottin asked Julie to review her latest version of the manuscript so she could then see if it was marketable. It is possible she waited to see if *Claire d'Albe,* coming out in May 1799, was a success before she attempted to interest her publisher in another manuscript. Cottin did not sign a contract with Maradan for publication of *Malvina* until September 1800 and it did not appear in print until January 1801, a full two years after André Cottin first saw it. Since the second novel was four times as long as the first, Maradan paid her four times the amount he had paid for *Claire d'Albe,* still cautious, most likely, because Cottin had yet to prove her staying power with the reading public. *Malvina* was published anonymously, with the author listed as "Mme ***, auteur de *Claire d'Albe*"; no published review or summary in 1800 revealed Cottin as the author. Only those within Cottin's circle of relatives and close associates knew.

But *Malvina* convinced Maradan that Sophie Cottin was a good risk; by June 1801, five months after the book first appeared, the first edition of 1,500 copies was sold out, and Maradan proposed to issue a second printing immediately, without changes or corrections to the original (*MC*, 29). A year later, in May 1802, when Maradan purchased the rights to *Amélie Mansfield*, which was the same length as *Malvina*, he was willing to pay Cottin 4,000 francs, over three times what he had paid for *Malvina*. Obviously, her stock had risen dramatically by that time, and the evidence indicates that it continued to rise throughout her lifetime.[1]

4
The Anger of *Amélie Mansfield*

During the first months of 1799, while waiting for her first novel to appear on Maradan's shelves, Cottin began a third novel. In a letter to André dated February 1799, she exclaimed: "Je veux écrire l'histoire de Charlotte Corday. . . . Oui, je veux l'écrire, à mon goût, à ma manière; peut-être la blâmera-t-on, peut-être sera-t-elle mauvaise, n'importe. Je ne sais écrire que d'après mes propres idées: s'il me fallait penser comme on me conseille, je ne saurais plus penser du tout" ["I want to write the story of Charlotte Corday. . . . Yes, I want to write it, according to my own taste, my own style; maybe people will criticize it, maybe it will be bad, it doesn't matter to me. I only know how to write according to my own ideas: if I had to think like others advise me to do, I wouldn't know how to think at all"] (*MC*, 322–23). Her attraction to Charlotte's story may have been based on her own feelings about the Revolution; perhaps she wanted to tell the story of a woman acting on her own, attempting to put a stop to what she perceived was an evil design. Even more specifically, Charlotte Corday was a man-killer, an angry woman who had stabbed a powerful man—Marat was, in many ways, the very icon of the Revolution—to death. Cottin told André: "Votre histoire de Charlotte m'a beaucoup intéressée. Je trouve, en effet, que c'est un sujet qui prête plus qu'un autre à exercer l'imagination" ["Your story about Charlotte interested me very much. I find, as a matter of fact, that it is a subject that, more than others, invites one to use one's imagination"] (322).[1] She admitted that, at the time, she could think of nothing else "capable de dissiper cet ennui profond de l'existence où je suis entraînée quelquefois" ["capable of dispelling this deep ennui about existence into which I fall sometimes"] (322). Writing, she said, helped her forget her ennui: "Je ne réponds pas que, dans mes moments de tristesse, je ne me sauve de moi-même au sein des malheurs de Charlotte" ["I do not deny that, in moments of sadness, I lose myself in the misfortunes of Charlotte"] (322). How could the story of this female assassin work as therapy for Sophie Cottin? Only a few pages of the Corday project survive, too little evidence upon which to found any solid conclusion. Cottin's next completed novel, however, *Amélie Mansfield,* did have as its heroine an angry young woman, disgusted and embittered by patriarchal society; in some ways, the same kind of anger that drove a Charlotte Corday to violence finds partial expression through Amélie, the most complex female character Cottin ever created.

Writing had evidently become an important source of income for Cottin. In her letter to Julie of December 1799, requesting that she review the *Malvina* manuscript, Cottin urged: "Hâte-toi de lire *Malvina,* pour que je puisse la corriger et voir ensuite à en tirer quelque chose" ["Hurry up and read *Malvina,* so I can correct it and then see if I can get something out of it"] (*MC*, 327). A clue as to the reason for the urgency is found in a succeeding line in the same letter: "Je suis attristée, effrayée de la manière dont l'argent se dissipe à Paris; les mémoires pleuvent" ["I am saddened, shocked at the way money vanishes into thin air in Paris; it is raining bills"] (327). Obviously, Cottin was counting on the sale of her second manuscript to help meet these financial obligations. In fact, Cottin had several different writing projects going on simultaneously in the years 1799 and 1800. While putting the final touches on *Malvina,* she was also working on *Amélie Mansfield* and evidently beginning research for a fourth novel, *Mathilde.* In a letter that Sykes dates sometime after May 1799 but before the end of 1800, Cottin asked André to send her several volumes of *La vie des saints* or anything like it: "j'ai un besoin très pressant de savoir positivement la vie qu'ils menaient dans les déserts de la Thébaïde, et surtout dans les cavernes du Liban" ["I have a very urgent need to know for sure the kind of life they led in the deserts of Thebes [Egypt], and especially in the caves of Lebanon"] (324). The material she gathered from André's books would provide the verisimilitude she needed to describe her heroine Mathilde's flight into the desert, only one of many episodes in what would turn out to be her longest novel. The urgency we feel in the wording of her request here suggests once again that Cottin felt a pressing need to get on with her writing; whether this urgency sprang from her financial situation or from her need to continue writing her stories, it is difficult to tell.

During the winter of 1800–1801, Julie was sent to Nice for health reasons. Indications in the correspondence suggest that Cottin took over sole responsibility for the girls in the absence of their mother. Probably because the girls were in school, Cottin moved to Paris to live once more in the Cottin residence on the chaussée d'Antin. In February 1801, she met Jean Devaines, a former bureaucrat under the ancien régime and litterateur of some reputation, who was approaching his sixty-sixth year. Critics—at least those who have found Devaines worth mentioning—have tried to understand the nature of the relationship between the two. Devaines's letters to Cottin reveal that he was greatly won over by her and pressed her to return his devotion—but to no avail. As she left Paris to return to Champlan in April, she let him know that she did not reciprocate his affection. She appeared to be puzzled by the fact that when she offered a man her friendship, he tended to want to develop the friendship into something else. Devaines explained to her: "C'est que, dès que vous croyez avoir rencontré une âme sur laquelle la vôtre puisse s'appuyer, vous épanchez une sensibilité si vive, votre affection se démontre avec tant d'abandon, toutes vos formes deviennent si tendres, qu'il n'est pas un homme qui ne vous livre, au même instant, toutes les facultés, dont l'ambition ne soit sur-le-champ de vous plaire, et qui ne mette pas le bonheur suprême à être aimé de vous" ["It is just that, as soon as you believe you have found a soul you can trust, you let loose such a strong flood of feelings, your affection shows itself without restraint, all your manners become so tender, that there is not a man alive who would not surrender to you, at that very instant, all his means, whose desire would not be to please you on the spot, and who would not consider it the greatest happiness to be loved by you"] (*MC*, 337).

Devaines continued to see Cottin, and she did not discourage his friendship. In fact, she relied on Devaines for his opinions about her new manuscript, *Amélie Mansfield*, which he was allowed to read and critique over a period of several months. He advised her to become her "plus sévère censeur" ["harshest critic"], to watch out for "les néologismes, les termes nouveaux, toute affectation" ["neologisms, new terms, all affectation"]: "La langue de Fénelon, de Voltaire, de Rousseau, voilà la seule bonne et qui soit digne de vous" ["The language of Fénelon, of Voltaire, of Rousseau, that is the only proper language and the only one worthy of you"] (*MC*, 336). Devaines suggested that, had he been around, the flaws people had found in *Malvina* would have been avoided.

Cottin ultimately became suspicious, however, of Devaines's critical judgment when it came to women writers. In a letter that appears never to have been sent to Devaines, Cottin explained that she had been reading some of his reviews of recent publications. His review of Madame de Genlis's novel was scathing because, Cottin maintained, the author was "vieille, laide, et intrigante" ["old, ugly, and scheming"]; on the other hand, a mediocre novel by, she assumed, a young, attractive woman was praised to the skies (*MC*, 343). Cottin had learned from this that she could no longer rely on getting the truth from him about her own writing, that, in fact, because of his attachment to her, he was the least reliable source for useful criticism: "Je vous crois flatteur avec les femmes, soit que leurs faibles talents ne vous semblent même pas dignes d'une critique, soit que, voulant leur plaire, vous croyez n'y réussir que par ce moyen. Lorsqu'il est question d'elles, on ne reconnaît plus ce goût pur, ce jugement exquis qui distingue tous vos autres ouvrages: non seulement vous manquez alors de sévérité, mais même de justesse et, qui plus est, de justice" ["I believe you flatter women, either because you do not consider their feeble talents worthy of criticism, or because, wanting to please them, you believe you can only succeed in this way. When it is a question of [women writers], one can no longer recognize the perfect taste, the elegant wisdom that are the hallmarks of all your other writings: you lack not only severity but sound judgment, too, and, even more importantly, fairness"] (343). All she asked of Devaines was to treat women equally, to subject their works to the same rigorous examination he used to evaluate male writers' works. As if to punish him for this hypocrisy, she concluded the letter with a vicious parting shot, the gist of which would not have escaped Devaines: "L'homme à cheveux blancs oublie, de son côté, que l'âge d'aimer n'a qu'un temps; il ose encore concevoir des désirs, et croit qu'en parlant d'amour, il inspire autre chose que la pitié" ["The old man forgets that the age of love comes but once; he still dares to fantasize, and believes that, in speaking of love, he inspires something other than merely pity"] (343). Perhaps Cottin felt she had allowed herself to become too angry and uncharacteristically vindictive and consequently did not send the letter; it nevertheless allows us to see that she wanted no preferential treatment or condescending attitudes from male critics. Her works deserved to be held to the same standards of quality applied in the case of a male writer.

As for contemporary male writers, Cottin reserved her highest praise for Chateaubriand. In April 1801, she wrote to Devaines describing her reaction to reading the latest best-seller, *Atala*: "Il y a là-dedans tout ce que j'aime: le désert, la mélancolie, la religion et l'amour" ["It has everything I love: the wilderness, melancholy, religion, and love"] (*MC*, 338). But, she admitted, it was mainly the local color and the thoughts scattered here and there that she admired most. The plot was not, in Cottin's opinion, the novel's strength, and the decision to have the narrator tell his own story in retrospect seriously weakens the novel's emotional impact because the reader already knows in advance that the narrator has survived the various adventures he is describing. Furthermore, she felt that Chateaubriand interrupted the narrative flow with far too many descriptions, causing the reader to become impatient and fatigued. In the end, though, she thought these weaknesses were compensated for by the text's powerful ideas: "J'aimais que quelqu'un eût pensé cela, et je goûtais un inexprimable plaisir à voir rendre, avec tant de charme, des réflexions dont le fond seul eût suffi pour me charmer" ["I was happy someone had thought these things, and I experienced an indescribable pleasure in seeing thoughts, the essence of which would have alone sufficed to please me, presented with so much charm"] (338–39). Particularly striking for her was Chateaubriand's ability to express a female's feelings: "Oh! qu'il a bien connu le coeur d'une femme passionnée, celui qui met dans la bouche d'Atala ce discours que la religion seule avait le droit d'interrompre, parce qu'elle seule pourrait être plus sublime que lui! Quand le délire de l'amour est porté au point de sacrifier l'éternité à son amant, et, aux portes de la mort, de pleurer de ne s'être pas perdue pour lui, il n'appartient qu'à Dieu de dire:—C'est mal; nous autres, faibles et légères créatures, pleurons et admirons" ["Oh! how he has understood well the heart of a woman in love, this author who causes Atala to utter words that religion alone had the right to interrupt, because only religion could be more sublime than her words! When love's delirium is such that, even at death's door, a woman is ready to sacrifice eternity for her lover and weeps because she has not given herself to him, only God has the right to say, 'This is wrong'; the rest of us, weak and frivolous creatures, let us weep and admire"] (338). Cottin appears almost ashamed to admit that she had been so moved by the text: "Peut-être ne durera-t-elle pas, mais, au premier moment, je ne sais point résister à l'espèce de magie qui est attachée pour moi à ces teintes mélancoliques, à ce profond amour de la solitude, à ce cri de la passion tempérée par la piété, qui répondent si bien à ce que j'ai de plus sensible dans le coeur" ["Maybe my first impression will not last, but, at present, I don't know how to resist the sort of magic associated for me with these melancholy hues, this profound love of solitude, this cry of passion tempered by religious devotion that echoes so closely my heart's most powerful feelings"] (339).

It is not surprising to find Cottin attracted by the conflict of passion and religion in Chateaubriand's work; it is after all, at its most fundamental, abstract level, this same tension between self-fulfillment and societal norms that functions as the mainspring for her own texts. The culturally subversive element she recognized in *Atala* drove her own writing. Even as she was revising *Malvina*, which emphasized duty and maternity over passion, Cottin was simultaneously writing the story of Amélie Mansfield, a female character whose disregard for cultural convention would cause Madame de Genlis to classify her as yet another Claire d'Albe. The simultaneous production of these different texts is striking: it is as if Cottin had two opposing forces tugging at her, unraveling one another and yet both needing to find expression in her writing. Perhaps the perfect emblem of the paradox of Cottin's heroines is Amélie Mansfield's face, which another character in the story describes as "mélange d'une pudeur souffrante et de la voluptueuse langueur" ["a mix of suffering modesty and sensual weakness"] (2:393). Amélie's story is one of an angry woman who attempts to isolate herself from patriarchal society, only to be drawn back into it with disastrous results.

Amélie Mansfield—an epistolary novel like the others before—was by far the most complex of Cottin's novels to date. The heroine, Amélie de Lunebourg, like Malvina, begins the novel as a widow and tells in retrospect the story of her first marriage. She recounts that she had been raised in an aristocratic family; her grandfather, the count of Woldemar, fearing that his descendants would dilute his proud bloodline by choosing to marry unworthy partners, had made a will in which he declared his grandson, Ernest de Woldemar, heir to his title and fortune on condition that he marry Amélie, his granddaughter and Ernest's cousin. Amélie, however, repulsed by the bad character of Ernest, had vowed never to marry him. She had been attracted instead to a commoner, Mansfield, a poet and musician. When Amélie's father and mother died, Ernest's mother, Madame de Woldemar, had attempted to get the family council to give her custody of Amélie, knowing that, if left to her own wishes, Amélie would not marry Ernest and the Woldemar family would lose the inheritance. Mansfield, seeing this, had pressed Amélie to marry him without anyone's permission; they had subsequently eloped to Prague and were married there. Amélie's bliss, however, had been short-lived; Mansfield, bored with her, began traveling away from home. Soon after a son was born, Amélie discovered evidence of her husband's infidelity. When her husband was killed in a duel over another woman, Amélie was left a widow at the age of twenty-two. As the novel regains the present, Amélie expresses her wish to have nothing more to do with marriage. Because she married below her station, her family wants nothing more to do with her.

When her late husband's uncle, M. Grandson, writes to offer to make her his heir if she will come live with him as his adopted daughter, in Bellinzonna, Switzerland, she accepts the proposal: "Flétrie par la douleur, éclairée par l'expérience, détrompée de l'amour, je ne désire plus que la solitude, la paix et l'amitié" ["Worn out by suffering, enlightened by experience, no longer deceived by love, I desire nothing more but solitude, peace, and friendship"] (2:301). She is happy being a daughter once again with a new "father," but the thought of being a wife again repulses her: "Moi, Amélie Mansfield, m'engager dans de nouveaux liens, quand tous mes souvenirs vivent encore; quand tous les mariages ne me présentent que l'image d'un ingrat et d'une victime; quand mon coeur, flétri par le chagrin, se sent dégoûté de tout, même du bonheur!" ["Me, Amélie Mansfield, commit myself to a new relationship when all my memories still live, when every marriage I see only shows me an ingrate and a victim, when my heart, withered by sorrow, is disgusted with everything, even happiness itself!"] (2:327). In a letter to her brother Albert, she describes her general aversion to men: "quand je réfléchis . . . au peu de vertus que j'ai trouvé dans ton sexe, je crois que je lui vouerais une sorte de mépris, si mon Albert n'en était pas" ["when I think of . . . the few virtues I have found in your sex, I believe I would have a sort of disdain for them all, if my Albert were not one of them"] (2:350). This pronouncement on men's frailties leads to a reiteration of her distrust of marriage: "c'est que mes infortunes passées m'ont inspiré un invincible éloignement pour le lien dont tu attends ta félicité, et que si j'avais le malheur d'aimer encore, je crois que je ne pourrais jamais me résoudre à former de nouveaux noeuds; il me semble qu'il y a moins de malheur à renoncer à l'objet de sa tendresse qu'à perdre son amour, et ce n'est pas dans la sainte union du mariage que l'amour se conserve; ma triste expérience . . . ne me l'[a] que trop prouvé" ["it's just that my past misfortunes have inspired an insurmountable revulsion in me for the relationship that you expect will bring you happiness, and if I had the unhappy lot of falling in love again, I believe I could never convince myself to marry again; it seems to me that it is easier to renounce the object of one's affection than to lose one's love, and love is not preserved in the holy bonds of matrimony; sad experience . . . has proven that to me only too well"] (2:352). When Albert protests against this condemnation of marriage, Amélie responds: "Je rejette le mariage, Albert, mais je crois que tout amour qui secoue son joug n'est ni pur ni heureux. Que ce lien sacré fasse donc le destin du monde; qu'il enchaîne tout ce qui aime, tout ce qui respire; qu'on voue au mépris la femme hardie qui oserait chercher le bonheur hors de lui; mais qu'il soit permis à l'infortunée qui fut sa victime d'y renoncer à jamais; et, si des sentiments trop tendres se réveillent dans son coeur, elle saura les reporter vers le ciel, et offrir à Dieu un amour qui n'a plus d'aliment sur la terre" ["I reject marriage, Albert, but I also believe that any love that tries to exist outside of marriage is neither virtuous nor happy. May this sacred bond be the fate of others; may it enslave all who love, all who breathe; may the bold woman who dares seek happiness outside marriage be condemned; but may it be permitted to the unfortunate woman who has been its victim to renounce it forever; and, if tender feelings awaken in her heart, she will know how to redirect them toward heaven and to offer God a love that cannot survive in the world"] (2:362).

Nowhere else in Cottin's texts do we find the institution of marriage so excoriated as here in *Amélie Mansfield*. Cottin's own marriage had not been difficult, but it had not lasted long; living with her cousin Julie had given her a true insider's perspective on the realities of most marriages in her day. Amélie's portrayal of marriage as nothing more than the binding together "of an ingrate and a victim" may very well reflect Cottin's own bitterness about arranged marriages, with their attendant mismatches in age and temperament.

In many ways, Amélie's words echo the rhetoric of Christian monasticism, and her move to Switzerland imitates a kind of monastic withdrawal from the world. By choosing to live with M. Grandson high in the Alps and dedicating herself to the rescue of lost or endangered travelers, Amélie effectually isolates herself from the world in order to pursue a higher spiritual goal. Here she is able to concentrate her energies on raising her child and demonstrating her courage and self-denial through service to others. The rise in elevation mirrors her determination to rise above the entanglements of human society, especially that of men and marriage, in order to purify her own life.

Unfortunately, the world once more intrudes: in a group of travelers she helps rescue from a storm is Ernest de Woldemar himself, who has made the trip with the express purpose of finding Amélie and taking revenge on her. He introduces himself under a false name, Henri Semler, and, since Amélie has not seen Ernest in fifteen years, the deception works. His grand design is to make her fall in love with him and then to reject her; he soon finds, however, that he is falling in love with her instead: "ce n'est point un ange; on est trop troublé auprès d'elle; mais, pour n'être qu'une femme, elle semble trop céleste et trop pure" ["she isn't an angel; she creates too much of a stir in your emotions when you're near her; but, for being only a woman, she seems too heavenly and too pure"] (2:353–54).

In a letter to his best friend, Adolphe, Ernest paints a word portrait of Amélie; she is charitable, generous, and simple, a peacemaker (2:355–56). As in *Claire d'Albe*, there is little mention of her physical attributes outside of "de grands yeux bleus, remplis de mélancolie, qu'elle élève habituellement vers le ciel, comme pour regarder sa patrie" ["large blue eyes, full of melancholy, that she lifts habitually toward the heavens, as if to gaze upon her homeland"] (2:354). His oath to worship no other woman but Amélie is based on the recognized superiority of her virtues: "j'ai été dire à cette terre qui la porte, à cet air qu'elle respire, à ces arbres qui la couvrent, à ce ciel qui la contemple que, tant qu'il restera une étincelle de vie dans mon coeur, je rendrai à cet unique assemblage de vertus, de grâces et de charmes, le culte sacré qui lui est dû" ["I have told this earth that bears her up, this air she breathes, these trees that shelter her, this heaven that watches over her that as long as a spark of life remains in my breast, I will pledge to this unique collection of virtue, grace, and charm the sacred devotion she deserves"] (2:358).

On the other hand, when he thinks of her as a mother, he is repulsed because her child Eugène is a physical representation of her former love. He swears he will never be a father to Mansfield's child. Increasingly, Ernest sees his relationship with Amélie as a struggle to win her away from her son. His extreme jealousy and hatred of Eugène are reiterated several times in this section of the text, perhaps to turn our affection as readers away from Ernest, making the obstruction to happiness for Amélie and Ernest very clear. When Amélie excuses herself to see to Eugène's needs, Ernest sarcastically begs forgiveness for having kept her away so long from her child, to which she energetically responds: "Oui, M. Semler, je vais le retrouver; en vain on tenterait de me le faire oublier: l'amitié n'y réussirait pas, et l'humeur encore moins. . . . [C]onçoit-on comment on peut en vouloir à une mère parce qu'elle chérit son enfant? . . . Ah! M. Semler! il est des sentiments auxquels on tient beaucoup sans doute; mais croyez qu'on les sacrifierait sans peine s'ils devaient nuire à d'autres plus anciens et bien sacrés" ["Yes, Mr. Semler, I am going to go find him; it is useless to try to make me forget him: friendship cannot do it, and anger even less. . . . [H]ow can one even imagine someone blaming a mother for loving her child? . . . Ah! Mr. Semler! there are no doubt feelings that one considers important; but you must understand that they would be easily sacrificed if they threatened older, more sacred ones"] (2:383–84). Ernest feels remorse for having said what he did to Amélie and tells Adolphe: "La meilleure des femmes peut-elle être mauvaise mère? et, s'il était possible que je lui devinsse assez cher pour lui faire oublier son fils, oserais-je l'estimer encore? oserais-je compter sur celle qui aurait sacrifié son premier devoir à l'amour?" ["Can the best of women be a bad mother? And if I were to become dear enough to her to make her forget her son, would I dare respect her still? Would I dare trust the woman who would have sacrificed her principal duty for love?"] (2:384).

Amélie, from her side, feels herself being drawn inexorably into a type of passion she has never known. She describes her struggle to Albert: "O mon frère! ceci finira mal pour moi: ce n'est plus cette faible préférence que m'inspira jadis M. Mansfield: c'est un sentiment dévorant qui m'égare, m'embrase, qui, dans tout l'univers, ne me laissant voir qu'un seul objet, et désirer qu'un seul bien, me fera mourir s'il s'éloigne, et lui appartenir s'il demeure. . . . [F]aible créature, qui n'as pas eu la force de te défendre contre l'amour" ["Oh, my dear brother! This will finish badly for me: this is no longer that weak attraction that I once felt for Mr. Mansfield: this is a consuming emotion, disorienting, burning, which, allowing me to see and desire, in all the universe, one thing alone, will kill me if he leaves, and make me give myself to him if he stays. . . . [F]eeble creature, who didn't have the strength to protect yourself from love"] (2:394–95). Amélie's confession that she has at last found love parallels in many ways the description Cottin used in *Claire d'Albe*, as this second Claire exclaims: "Je me sens si heureuse! . . . oh! ces instants d'ineffables délices, quelle place ils tiennent dans la vie! eux seuls font vivre: tout le reste n'est rien" ["I feel so happy! . . . [O]h! these moments of ineffable delights, how important they are in life! They alone make you live: everything else is nothing"] (2:398).

She imagines her brother's gaze, which for her duplicates that of God: "Ô Albert! ne me regarde pas ainsi; mon frère, aie compassion de ta soeur; elle ne se dissimule pas ses fautes; elle prévoit tous tes reproches; elle voudrait être digne de toi, elle ne le peut plus: une force inconnue l'entraîne, un esprit de vertige et d'erreur semble répandu autour d'elle; n'est-elle pas prête à donner sa main et à livrer son sort, sa volonté et sa vie, à l'ennemi de son enfant?" ["Oh, Albert! Don't look at me that way; dear brother, have compassion on your sister; she doesn't hide her sins; she foresees all your reproaches; she would like to be worthy of you, she can no longer be: an unknown force is carrying her along, a feeling of giddiness and error seems to encircle her; is she not on the verge of giving her hand and yielding her future, her will, and her life to the enemy of her child?"] (2:395). Almost echoing the words of Chateaubriand's Atala, Amélie admits that her passion for Ernest—whom she stills knows only by his false name Henri—is now stronger than her devotion to God: "je sens, en frémissant, que je crains moins de me perdre, que d'être sauvée par son indifférence. A ce mot, je tombe à genoux devant ce ciel que j'offense, devant toi, mon vertueux frère, qui dois rougir de me nommer ta soeur: je voudrais que la terre m'engloutît" ["Trembling, I feel that being damned is less frightening than being saved because of [Ernest's] indifference. At these words, I fall to my knees before the very divinity I am offending, before you, my virtuous brother, who must blush to call me his sister: I want the earth to swallow me up"] (2:396).

Ernest, meanwhile, feels the eyes of his mother on him. He has not seen her for ten years, and she writes to tell him that her increasingly bad health is the result of his long absence. She warns him that if he has made a bad choice and become unworthy of being her son, it will kill her. Fearing her disapproval, Ernest informs Amélie he cannot marry her; when Grandson learns of this, he becomes furious and chases Ernest from the house. Insisting on seeing Amélie one last time, Ernest—still posing as Henri—writes her a note laden with hidden meaning: "Amélie, nous fûmes, dès le berceau, destinés l'un à l'autre, et notre sort voulait que nous fussions unis. Je peux mourir ce soir, mais, je le jure, je ne mourrai point sans avoir accompli notre sort" ["Amélie, from the cradle, we were meant for each other, and fate wanted us to be as one. I can die this evening, but I swear I will not die without fulfilling our destiny"] (2:408). He threatens to kill himself if she will not see him; Amélie concedes and gives him permission to visit her one last time on her balcony at midnight. She writes a desperate note to her brother: "Dieu seul pourrait me secourir, et je ne puis prier.... [J]e t'appelle, et tu ne m'entends pas; je t'appelle.... O mon frère! serait-ce là le dernier effort de la vertu de ta malheureuse soeur?" ["Only God could save me, and I cannot bring myself to pray.... I call out for you, and you don't hear me; I am calling out for you.... Oh, dear brother! Could this be the last effort your unfortunate sister's virtue will make?"] (2:417).

In Amélie, Cottin shows us a heroine who, true to her word, does not need the cultural institution of marriage to celebrate her love and who declares herself free of such necessities. When Ernest arrives, the two swear to one another that they will never marry anyone else. During the time he spends in her bedroom that night, they start calling one another *épouse* and *époux*; this is only a marriage of wishful dreams, but it is consummated just as if they had been joined together in a ceremony. As readers, we recognize that Amélie is a virtuous woman who, having been victimized earlier in her life in a contract sanctioned by society, now chooses to act out her desires according to her own conception of happiness. Like Claire before her, Amélie dares to decide for herself what she needs for completion or plenitude.

In this, however, she will be deceived. As dawn breaks, Amélie wants to know why Ernest had refused her uncle's offer to have them married. She insists on knowing his name, but he is sure that if he tells her his real name, it will kill her. He lies a second time, telling her that his name is Adolphe; Amélie recognizes it as the name of Ernest de Woldemar's best friend and consequently faints. The commotion brings her servants; Ernest flees through the balcony and, when he is about to be discovered by Grandson, dives into the lake and reaches his boat. In a letter, he asks Amélie to run away with him: "[F]uyons au bord de l'univers; allons consacrer nos noeuds sous un autre hémisphère; nous serons tout l'un pour l'autre, et nous oublierons ce monde où il faut dissimuler, souffrir, être oppresseur ou victime" ["[L]et us flee to the very edge of the universe; let us sanctify our vows in another hemisphere; we will live only for one another and forget this world where one must lie and suffer and be either the oppressor or the victim"] (2:422). Even while saying this, he claims her surrender to him has made him "le maître d'Amélie" ["Amélie's master"] and that she no longer has the right to refuse him (2:422).

But Amélie will not run away with him: "Ô mon Adolphe! dans l'abîme où l'amour m'a plongée, tu t'étonneras peut-être de m'entendre encore parler de devoirs; mais écoute: si j'ai pu les trahir pour toi, je ne me résoudrai jamais à te les voir méconnaître; et du moins, en manquant à la vertu, je n'aurai fait tort qu'à moi" ["Oh, Adolphe! in the inferno into which love has plunged me, you will perhaps be surprised to hear me speak once again of duty; but listen: even if I was capable of failing my duty because of you, I will never bring myself to let you belittle it; and at least, in failing to be virtuous, I will have hurt only myself"] (2:423). He answers, much as Frédéric in *Claire d'Albe* had done: "toi, âme de ma vie, que jamais l'ombre d'un repentir n'arrive jusqu'à ton coeur, et garde-toi de croire que Dieu puisse nous faire un crime sur la terre de cet amour qui doit être notre récompense dans le ciel" ["love of my life, may the least bit of repentance never enter your heart, and don't let yourself believe that God could make this love that is to be our heavenly reward a transgression for us while on earth"] (2:426).

Ernest's resolve to do everything necessary to have Amélie as his wife, including revealing his true identity to her, does not hold up when, upon his return to Woldemar, he once again faces his mother. Day after day, Ernest delays the revelation of his secret, always finding some excuse not to tell her. The narrative style here—reminiscent of Wagner's tension-building chromaticism—defers gratification or resolution until the exhausted reader arrives at the final scene with nerves stretched to the snapping point. Ernest speaks incessantly of revealing his plan to his mother, but something invariably impedes the revelation. The mother's hatred for Amélie is made excruciatingly clear through episode after episode—fifteen pages of text, to be exact—while Ernest is supposedly getting up the courage to reveal his secret. "Demain est le jour fixé pour m'expliquer avec ma mère" ["Tomorrow is the day I have set to explain everything to my mother"], he writes to his friend, "demain je connaîtrai mon sort, et tout sera fini" ["tomorrow I will know my fate, and all will be finished"] (2:444). But tomorrow comes and goes many times without the revelation being made.

Finally, the secret is discovered when his mother finds him talking to Amélie's portrait; Mme. de Woldemar is outraged that her son would want to marry the very woman who had once chosen a commoner over himself. She declares that he must choose: "Vivre pour Amélie! c'est donner la mort à votre mère: choisissez, mon fils" ["To live for Amélie is to kill your mother: choose, my son"] (2:450). In one scene, Mme. de Woldemar tells Ernest that Amélie's sin can never be erased; the sin she refers to, however, is not the immoral conduct of which they are guilty but rather Amélie's marriage to a commoner: "sa conduite l'a souillée d'une tache indélébile qu'aucune puissance de la terre ne peut effacer" ["her conduct has stained her with an indelible stain that no earthly power can erase"] (2:459). Mme. de Woldemar warns Ernest that if he marries Amélie, "les hommes de la plus basse extraction pourront vous dire: 'Je vaux mieux que toi, car je suis resté dans le rang où le ciel m'a placé; mais toi, c'est par ta faute que tu as perdu le tien'" ["men of the lowest extraction will be able to say to you: 'I am better than you, because I stayed where heaven placed me; but you, through your own mistakes, have lost your station'"] (2:459). When Ernest persists in his allegiance to Amélie in spite of his mother's command to forget her, Mme. de Woldemar faints. During the twenty-four hours his mother is unconscious, Ernest says, "l'image d'Amélie ne s'est pas présentée une seule fois à ma pensée" ["Amélie's face did not come to my mind a single time"], a fact he considers a telling sign (2:461).

When his mother revives, she asks for him. In his letter to Adolphe, Ernest confesses, "j'ai senti qu'une mère qu'on vient d'assassiner, et qui vous bénit encore, avait plus de puissance sur le coeur que l'amour même" ["I realized that a mother whom you had just killed and who still pronounces a blessing on you had more power over the heart than love itself"] (2:461). His mother, claiming that she will die if he does not give up Amélie, finally convinces him to obey her. Ernest, who has never revealed his name to Amélie, now asks Adolphe to take all his letters to Amélie and tell her that he has died. His self-confessed struggle is "contre l'ambition et la volonté de sa mère" ["against the ambition and will of his mother"], so it is not duty alone that makes him hesitate; there is also the question of his class and his future (2:453). Ernest knows that to disobey his mother is to consign himself to "errant dans les terres étrangères, et portant partout le remords de l'avoir offensée" ["wandering in strange lands and carrying everywhere the remorse of having trespassed against her"] (2:444). In other words, he will be cut off from the family fortune.

Ernest begins having nightmares of Amélie in which she appears pleading, desperate, and near death. Thinking that she may already be dead, he stabs himself in the presence of his mother. Horrified, Mme. de Woldemar consents to his marrying Amélie but only after he spends the next few months at the emperor's court in Vienna; if, at the end of that period, he has not changed his mind about Amélie, she will not stand in his way: "Alors mon fils, disant un éternel adieu au monde, à la cour, à votre patrie, dont vous étiez destiné à faire l'ornement, vous irez vous ensevelir dans vos montagnes, pour y traîner vos déplorables jours avec celle à qui vous aurez tout sacrifié; votre mère ne s'y opposera plus" ["Then, my son, saying an eternal farewell to the world, to the court, to your fatherland in which you were destined to become a shining star, you will bury yourself in the mountains, there to lead a lamentable life with the woman for whom you have sacrificed everything; your mother will no longer oppose it"] (2:475). Ernest is overjoyed; he can at last reveal his true identity to Amélie. He writes her a letter, exclaiming: "Avenir enchanteur! retrouver ton regard, ton sourire, te presser sur mon coeur, te posséder à jamais, voilà donc quel sera mon sort! tu m'aimes et tu seras à moi" ["Wonderful prospect! to see your face again, your smile, to hold you to my breast, to possess you forever, this will be my lot! You love me and you will be mine"] (2:485).

Amélie, however, has already learned his true identity, thanks to a letter written by Ernest's sister to Albert but intercepted by Amélie. Outraged, she proclaims: "je fuis, je renonce à vous, je renonce à tout; je hais un monde où il se trouve de pareilles douleurs et de telles perfidies" ["I am running away, I renounce you, I renounce everything; I hate a world in which there is such sorrow and treachery"] (2:489). Amélie leaves the house of her adoptive uncle, asking that he take care of her son in her absence. She does not reveal her plans or destination, but at this point, the story shifts to a different narrative form, the personal journal, allowing the reader to see into the private thoughts of the heroine. Beginning it, Amélie explains, "je veux laisser un journal; j'y inscrirai toutes mes pensées, toutes mes actions" ["I want to leave a diary; I will write all my thoughts in it, all my actions"] (2:489). The journal reveals that she is pregnant; desperate and contemplating suicide, she has abandoned her son in order to find her lover: "Tandis que je descendais la montagne, l'ombre plaintive de mon fils errait autour de moi; je croyais l'entendre gémir: 'Laisse-moi, m'écriai-je, laisse-moi aller chercher le père de cette autre victime'" ["As I descended the mountain, my son's plaintive ghost dogged my heels; I thought I heard him wailing: 'Leave me alone,' I cried, 'let me find the father of this other victim'"] (2:491–92). Here again, we find the word "victim," this time applied to the unborn child she carries. Amélie has already claimed that a woman is victimized in marriage; now the victims have tripled in number because the living and the unborn children as well as the abandoned woman herself suffer the consequences of the lover's perfidy.

It becomes increasingly evident as the story progresses that the search for Ernest can only end in tragedy. A premonition drives Amélie on to Dresden; it is now the end of August and she is over three months along in her pregnancy. She begins to suspect that her worst enemy may be the father of the child she is carrying: "je ne crois plus aux serments, je ne crois plus à la parole d'aucun homme; il n'y a dans leur coeur que trahison, duplicité, mensonge" ["I don't believe in vows anymore, I don't believe the word of any man anymore; there is nothing but betrayal, duplicity, and lies in their hearts"] (2:502). Amélie wants to go to Woldemar, find Ernest, and "expirer à ses yeux sur la tombe de mon père" ["die on my father's grave while he watches"] (2:505). Death on the father's tomb connects Amélie once more with Claire d'Albe; like Claire, Amélie wishes for death, but this time death will allow the heroine to escape both Father and Lover, the first because she is so desperately ashamed of her lost innocence, and the second because she despises him as a deceiver.

Ernest, however, is not at Woldemar; he has been taken to Vienna by his mother, Amélie is told, to find him a wife. And so Amélie too makes her way to Vienna where, during a masked ball, she observes Ernest talking with Blanche, his cousin, and misreads the gestures. Amélie scribbles a note, hands it to Ernest without a word, and leaves. The note says she has seen his betrayal and that if he wants to find her, she will be in the river. Ernest rushes to the river, enlisting the help of those nearby to search for a woman wearing a mask. Someone shouts they have found a body on the bank. Ernest runs to the crowd, takes off the mask, recognizes Amélie, believes she is dead, and faints beside her body.

In the original version of this story, Cottin had indeed made her heroine attempt suicide. The fever that comes as a result of the attempt ultimately takes her life as well as that of her unborn child. In subsequent editions, Cottin revised the plot: instead of throwing herself into the river, Amélie faints on the bank, unable to bring herself to commit suicide which, she says, would have offended God (*MC*, 413). The revision indicates that Cottin may have realized that her reading audience would sympathize more with her heroine if Amélie remained a total victim and did not become responsible for her own death. The original version, on the other hand, shows us a woman who defies both God and society in deciding to kill herself; she acts as she herself and she alone judges best. In many ways, the original version is more consistent with the heroine Cottin had created up to this point in the narrative, a heroine who bears an interesting resemblance to the Atala she admitted to admiring.

Amélie is taken inside; though she is very sick, she will not let the doctor touch her. When Mme. de Woldemar comes at last to see Amélie, she accuses Amélie of trying to ruin the good name of her house and her son and asks her to make the sacrifice that will guarantee Ernest a happy future. Ernest maintains that he and Amélie already belong to one another, that Amélie is already his wife. Mme. de Woldemar pushes Amélie to say the same; all Amélie can say, however, is that she belongs to Ernest but is not his legal wife. Then the fatal words come out: "le ciel sait que, si j'avais cru faire ton bonheur en dévoilant ma honte, je ne l'aurais pas caché si longtemps" ["the heavens know that, if I had believed I would make him happy in revealing my shame, I would not have hidden it for so long"] (2:537). Blanche describes the effect Amélie's confession has on the people in the room: "A cet aveu, ma mère s'est couvert le visage, mon père s'est levé, la baronne a paru satisfaite, et j'ai laissé échapper un cri de douleur" ["At this confession, my mother covered her face, my father rose to his feet, the baroness seemed satisfied, and I cried out in sorrow"] (2:537). Ernest is thrilled with the news. Mme. de Woldemar refuses to give her consent to a marriage, but she says she will abandon Ernest, leave him the house, and let him do whatever he will, and she will enter a convent.

In a letter to Adolphe, Mme. de Woldemar appears to have softened; she fears for the life of Amélie and says that if there is a real danger she will give in. Albert arrives in Vienna with M. Grandson and Amélie's son. Albert knows his sister too well: "Amélie n'endurera pas un regard de mépris; elle croit que tout ce qui l'entoure a le droit de la faire rougir; et du moment qu'elle a dévoilé sa honte, elle était sûre de mourir" ["Amélie will not endure a look of contempt; she believes that everyone around her has the right to make her blush; and from the moment she revealed her shame, she was sure to die"] (2:537). Ernest too is now very ill with a fever but will not do anything for himself; he and Amélie appear to have resolved to die together.

Close to death, Amélie says she cannot hope for a happy afterlife: "Que suis-je? une pauvre créature bien criminelle: je n'ai pas su résister à l'amour, et j'ai répandu sur toute ma famille l'opprobre et la douleur" ["What am I? a poor guilty creature: I couldn't resist love, and I have brought disgrace and suffering on all my family"] (2:544). Speaking of Ernest's mother, she instructs him: "dites-lui bien que ce n'est pas sa rigueur qui me tue, le coup part de plus loin, et si je n'eusse pas été coupable, j'aurais supporté mes adversités; mais vivre sans innocence, avoir perdu le contentement de moi-même et l'estime d'Albert, c'était trop pour moi. . . . Ô Ernest! pardonne si je n'ai pu me consoler de t'avoir tout sacrifié; mais la vertu ne m'était pas moins chère que ton amour; et, privée de l'une ou de l'autre, il fallait mourir" ["tell her that it is not her severity that is killing me, the blow comes from much farther away, and if I hadn't been guilty, I would have endured my adversity; but to live without virtue, to have lost my self-respect and the respect of Albert, was too much for me. . . . Oh, Ernest! forgive me if I cannot console myself with the idea of having sacrificed everything for you; but virtue was no less dear to me than your love; and, deprived of either one or the other, I had to die"] (2:547–48).

This heroine dies with an unborn child in her womb, her death essentially self-inflicted. It is clear that Amélie never intends to give birth to an illegitimate child; she cannot bear the shame. Amélie is incomplete without her virtue; having lost it, there remains no other compelling reason, no duty or obligation, to continue living. She will abandon her only living child to others to raise and take the life of her unborn child in taking her own. As in *Claire d'Albe*, a heroine decides that maternity and maternal duties are insufficient for complete happiness but this time, rather than dying because she cannot have her lover, the heroine dies because she cannot live without self-respect. Amélie cannot love herself anymore: "vivre sans innocence, avoir perdu le contentement de moi-même . . . c'était trop pour moi" ["to live without virtue, to have lost my self-respect . . . was too much for me"] (2:548). This may be a different approach to female plenitude for Sophie Cottin: though pregnant—*pleine*—her heroine determines that she has lost an essential part of her identity, with no hope of restoration or redemption of that essential part. As a consequence of that loss, Amélie erases herself from existence; the text tells us that the orphan she leaves with her death is "la seule image qui restât d'elle sur la terre" ["the only image of her that remained behind on earth"] (2:560).

"Tout être seul n'est pas heureux" ["Anyone who is alone is unhappy"], Cottin once wrote (*MC*, 350). The orphan is an image of incompletion; he lacks something—the parental presence that helps establish identity and place. The orphan child also has no protector and is thus placed in harm's way to become a victim of larger, more powerful forces than he. The absent Father thrust Amélie into a world where she became a victim. Amélie subsequently lost all faith in patriarchal society and expressed an intense anger toward it. Like an orphan, she felt herself left at the mercy of forces she could not control. Her solution was to isolate herself from that society, hiding away in the Alps. When she leaves this safe haven, the results are disastrous.

Amélie is by far Sophie Cottin's angriest heroine; in some ways, perhaps, she carries Cottin's own anger as a woman who felt herself a victim. Anger, as we have seen, is one of the typical reactions of the infertile individual, the result of feeling that one is at the mercy of forces beyond one's control. Societal pressures can intensify the anger, and so the urge to isolate oneself from society becomes very strong. The sufferer tries to find ways of escaping from more potential pain. Cottin's preference for the life at Champlan, associating only with a select entourage of family and friends, was very likely linked to her self-perceived defectiveness; isolation helped her avoid having to talk about her condition or to defend her life choices. Her heroine Amélie Mansfield exhibits a similar dislike for human company.

In all three of the novels we have studied thus far, strong feelings of guilt have driven the heroine to the point where she seeks death. And in all three cases, the heroine feels she has been both the victim and perpetrator of wrong. Here again, the fictional emblem of victim/criminal may point toward Cottin's own struggle, since those who are infertile, even in modern society, as we have already learned, harbor feelings that they must have done something wrong to deserve the punishment of infertility. They are likely to feel "unworthy and incapable in every sector."[2] Childlessness can, in the real world, lead to "loss of faith, loss of power, [and] loss of dreams."[3] The urge to seek a way to "atone" and thereby to lessen guilt becomes very strong. Interestingly, much of this appears to have found its way into Cottin's fictional world: her three guilt-ridden heroines—Claire, Malvina, and Amélie—all allow themselves to slide slowly from existence as their atonement of choice.

Cottin sold the manuscript of *Amélie Mansfield* to Maradan in May 1802; the novel appeared in bookstores in late December 1802 or January 1803. Like her two previous novels, it was published without her name but the connection with the two other successful works was evident in the wording on the title page: "Madame ***, author of *Claire d'Albe* and *Malvina*."

As she completed *Amélie Mansfield,* Cottin was entering a

period of religious revival in her personal life. The causes of this may be difficult to determine, but one of its consequences is clear: never again would Amélie's or Claire's type appear as the central character of one of her novels. From this point on, Cottin saw herself increasingly as a defender of the faith. Perhaps it was part of the atonement process for her. Events over the next two years would convince her that she had indeed chosen wisely.

5
Mathilde and the Miracle of Bagnères

Bagnères-de-Bigorre, situated in the foothills of the French Pyrenees at an altitude of 1,835 feet, has for centuries attracted those seeking healing to its famous mineral hot springs. The formerly small village—now become a town—sits nestled in the valley of the Adour river; everywhere, fountains spout the water from which the site has derived its fame. Sophie Cottin was well acquainted with Bagnères and the surrounding region, the result of trips made to the area in her youth. When Devaines died in March 1803, Cottin's thoughts apparently turned to the possibility of a pilgrimage of sorts she would make to Bagnères: "j'ai besoin de distractions. Continuer ma même vie, et la continuer sans lui [Devaines], me jetterait, j'en suis sûre, dans une mélancolie qui dégénérerait en dégoût universel, triste état auquel je ne suis que trop disposée. . . . [J]'ai donc saisi avidement l'idée d'aller à Tonneins avec M. Verdier, et de là aux Pyrénées" ["I need a diversion. To continue my same life and to continue it without [Devaines] would, I am sure, throw me into a melancholy state that would degenerate into a general disgust, a sad state to which I am only too much inclined. . . . I have therefore eagerly seized upon the idea of going to Tonneins with M. Verdier, and from there to the Pyrenees"] (*MC*, 353).

In a letter dated May 1803 written to an unknown male friend, Cottin referred to Devaines as a lost "father" whose wise counsel had guided her along the path of reason and whose friendship had saved her from her own ennui. Now, she wrote, "que je suis profondément dégoûtée de tous ces êtres avec qui il faut vivre, et quel mépris amer je ne puis m'empêcher de concevoir pour ceux qui ont osé profaner par un soupçon la pureté d'une si sainte amitié!" ["how thoroughly disgusted I am with all these people with whom one must live, and what bitter contempt I cannot help feeling for those who dared profane the purity of such a sacred friendship with their suspicions!"] (*MC*, 353). Devaines had come along at a

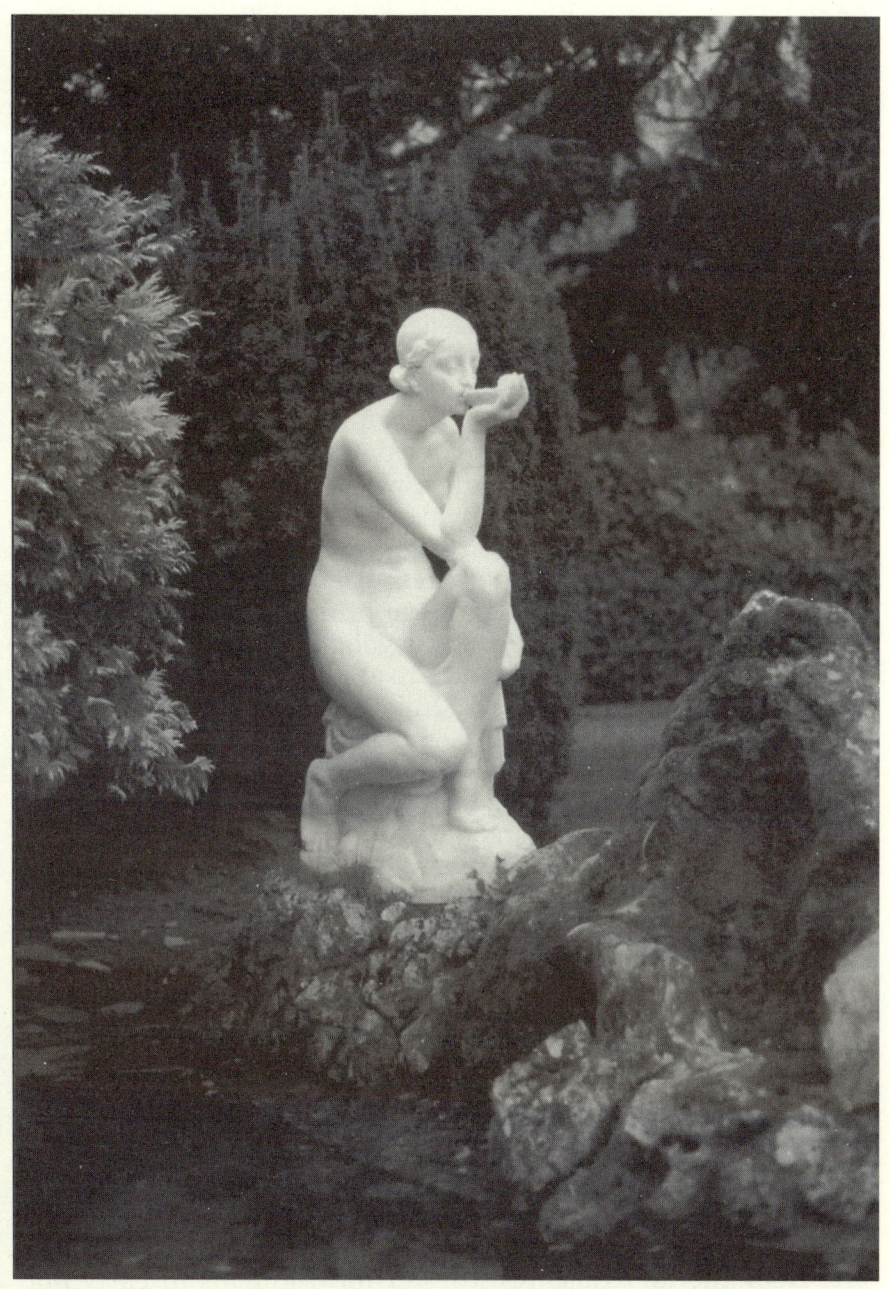

La Jouvence (the Fountain of Youth) by Popineau, 1934, Place des Thermes, Bagnères-de-Bigorre, France. Photograph Michael J. Call.

time when she thought she was losing Julie: "Hélas! cette amitié ne s'était nourrie que de douleurs, et c'est peut-être ce qui me l'avait rendue si chère. Elle est née au moment où des chagrins m'accablaient, où je croyais ne plus voir mon amie [Julie], et où l'intérêt de ses filles m'imposait le désir de vivre" ["Alas! this friendship was fed only by pain, and that is perhaps what made it so dear to me. It was born at a time when I was overcome by grief, when I did not believe I would see my friend [Julie] again, and when, for her daughters' sake, I was forced to want to live"] (353–54). In fact, in Julie's absence, Cottin assumed the role of full-time mother to Julie's daughters; in a letter to Mme. de Pastoret during this period, she referred to them as "mes trois enfants" ["my three children"] (*UO*, 142).

The Pyrenees offered curative waters as well as a temperate climate, and Cottin was concerned with Julie's long-term health problems. The two women apparently decided they would try Bagnères to see if Julie's health improved and make a decision about a longer stay later. The trip south would be made ostensibly for Julie's sake. The pilgrimage promised healing on more than one level, however. Cottin was going through a religious revival of sorts, perhaps in part the result of Devaines's death but also because of the near loss of Julie. In a letter dated from the days of preparation for the trip, she exhorted a friend: "Ah! que vous puissiez revenir à la seule vérité qui soit au monde, à la religion, à cette religion divine, évangélique, toute d'indulgence et d'amour, qui encourage le repentir, réprime l'orgueil, console le malheureux, soutient le misérable, et remplit le coeur des heureux de l'image de leurs frères souffrants et du désir de les soulager" ["Oh! if you could return to the only truth in the world, to religion, to that divine religion, evangelical, full of indulgence and love, which encourages repentance, suppresses pride, consoles those who are unhappy, buoys up those in misery, and fills the hearts of the fortunate with the image of their suffering brothers and the desire to help them"] (*MC*, 354). There is little evidence of this type of religious fervor in her correspondence up to this date and so it appears that the trip to the Pyrenees held symbolic significance as Cottin felt herself returning to her spiritual roots as well as to her geographical homeland.

Traveling with Julie, her husband, and the two eldest daughters, Delphine and Elisa, Cottin left for Tonneins in early May 1803. Mathilde, the third daughter, was placed in a boarding school in Versailles, probably so as to not break up her education with a long vacation. The little group stayed in Tonneins for approximately two months, during which Julie and Cottin rejoiced in rediscovering the places they had known as children where their friendship began. Delphine and Elisa, for their part, made a good impression on the local crowd, according to reports Cottin sent to friends back in Paris.

In late July 1803, the women and children moved on to Bagnères-de-Bigorre where they rented an apartment in a house owned and inhabited by François-Marie Soubies, a local government official. Soubies's unmarried sister, Fanny, who also lived in the home, became in time Cottin's close friend. Describing her feelings about the rediscovery of the Pyrenees in a letter to her brother-in-law, Cottin rhapsodized:

> J'ai éprouvé un plaisir si doux et si vif à revoir mes belles montagnes, mes eaux si limpides, mes vertes et fraîches prairies, qu'il me serait impossible de ne pas vous en dire quelque chose; l'effet que produit sur moi la vue de ce pays-ci est bizarre et, quoique toujours le même, il me surprend toujours. . . . Il n'y a point de quartiers ici d'où on ne respire la fraîcheur des eaux, d'où on n'entende leur doux murmure; il n'y a point de cabane dans les environs dont on n'ambitionne de faire sa demeure, et on ne peut aller boire les eaux et prendre les bains qu'en traversant des lieux enchantés, de véritables paradis terrestres.
>
> [I felt such a sweet and intense pleasure in seeing my beautiful mountains again, my waters so clear, my fresh, green fields, that it would be impossible for me not to tell you something about it; the effect that seeing this countryside produces in me is strange and, though always the same, it always surprises me. . . . In every part of town here you breathe in the freshness of the water, you hear its soft murmuring; there isn't a house in the area in which you wouldn't want to live, and you can't go to drink the water or bathe at the spa without crossing an enchanted land, true paradises on earth.] (*UO*, 150–51).

The walk from town to Cottin's favorite site, the Salut hot springs, followed a small stream through a delightful wooded area. Even today the visitor to Bagnères can retrace the very route leading to the baths that Cottin herself took.

A typical day for Cottin at Bagnères included many and varied activities, the principal of which were writing and tutoring. She described her daily schedule as follows:

> Je me lève de très bonne heure; jusqu'à l'heure du déjeuner je me mets à écrire; à neuf heures on m'annonce que le café est prêt, les enfants arrivent, Julie un peu plus tard, enfin tout se réunit. Après le

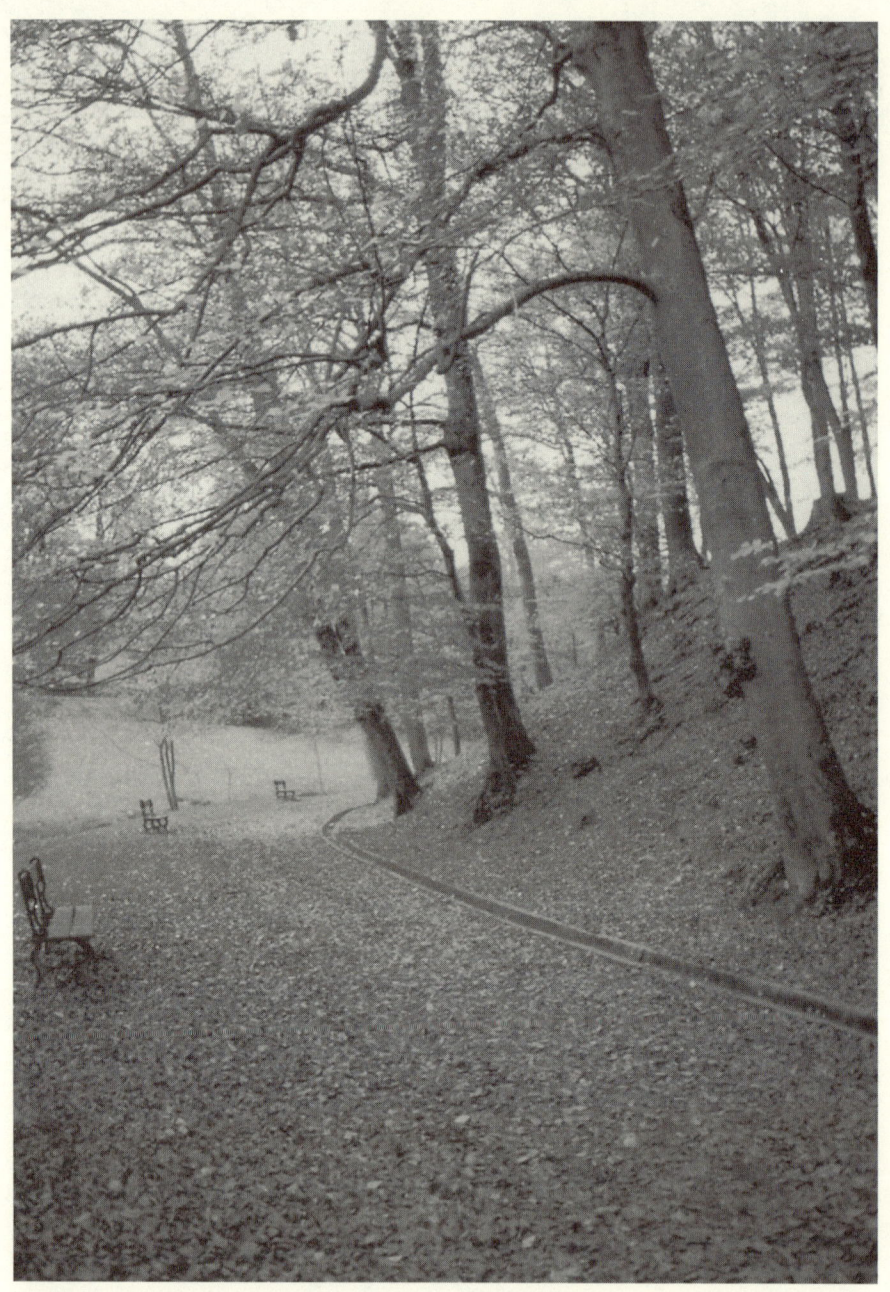

Path in the Vallon du Salut, leading from Bagnères to the spa Cottin frequented known as the Thermes du Salut, Bagnères-de-Bigorre, France. Photograph Michael J. Call.

5: *MATHILDE* AND THE MIRACLE OF BAGNÈRES

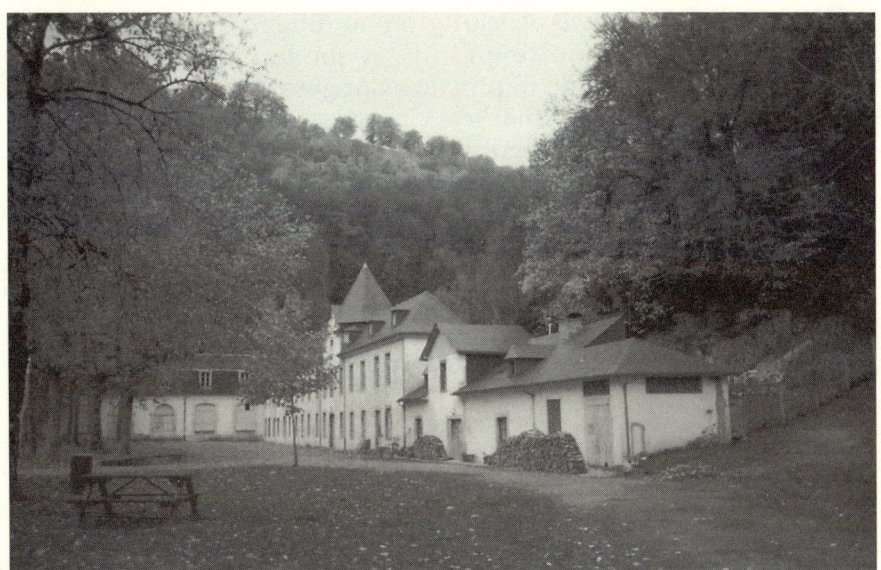

Les Thermes du Salut, Bagnères-de-Bigorre, France. Photograph Michael J. Call.

repas, l'heure des leçons sonne, j'en donne d'anglais et de musique, Julie de plus utiles encore; elles durent jusqu'au dîner, excepté quand le soleil vient au nom de ses brillants rayons nous jurer de les interrompre pour aller le voir de plus près; il est vrai que nous n'obéissons pas à ses douces prières. Après le dîner, Julie coud, tricote, raccommode, lit avec ses enfants, moi j'écris jusqu'à sept heures et demie.

[I get up very early; I write until breakfast; at 9:00 they announce the coffee is ready, the children arrive, Julie a little later, finally everyone is there. After the meal, the time for lessons comes, I teach English and music, Julie even more practical lessons; these last until dinner, except when the sun comes with its warm rays, urging us to leave lessons behind and come outside; it's true we don't always obey its gentle prodding. After dinner, Julie sews, knits, darns, or reads to the children; myself I write until 7:30.] (*UO*, 209–10)

At 8:00, assembled in the salon, the women and their gentlemen friends—among them Hyacinthe Azaïs, tutor of the Soubies children—amused themselves with music; Delphine played the piano, Azaïs, an accomplished musician, accompanied her on the violin, and Eliza sang. At 9:00 the group dined, and by 11:00, everyone was in bed (211). Some days, Cottin would leave the house in the early morning and spend the entire day walking, not returning until dinner time (242).

The novel Cottin was working on so diligently was *Mathilde*, "un ouvrage qui démontre qu'il n'y a que la religion chrétienne qui puisse préserver une femme des dangers de la séduction" ["a work that demonstrates that the Christian religion is the only religion capable of protecting a woman from the dangers of seduction"] (*UO*, 196). She admitted to her brother-in-law André that the people of Bagnères found it hard to believe she was the same woman who had written the novels they had read:

> Mais, tandis que mes lettres me peignaient à vous une femme exaltée "qui rêve des histoires sur le bord des torrents" et "qui est en prière dans les cavernes sombres," les personnes qui me voyaient habituellement à Bagnères me peignaient comme une femme pleine de raison, de sens et de réserve. Elles ne pouvaient même assez s'étonner de trouver ces espèces de qualités-là dans la même femme qui avait fait les ouvrages qu'elles avaient lus. Que conclure de tout cela, mon frère, et comment arrangez-vous tant de contrastes? Hé quoi, vous est-il si difficile de joindre un peu de raison à l'imagination que vous m'accordez et de croire que la première seule me dirige dans les choses graves, tandis que je ne suis sous l'empire de l'autre que quand je m'amuse à rêver ou à écrire?

> While my letters led you to see me as an impassioned woman "who dreams up stories on the banks of raging rivers" and "prays in dark caves," the people in Bagnères who saw me daily thought of me as a reasonable, sensible, and reserved woman. They could hardly get over seeing these traits in the same woman who had written the works they had read. What can one conclude from all this, my brother, and how do you reconcile such contrasts? Well, is it so hard for you to couple a little reason to the imagination you grant me and to believe that the former directs me in serious things, while I am only under the sway of the latter when I entertain myself by dreaming or writing?] (197–98)

By September, Cottin could report to her friend Madame de Pastoret that Julie was already feeling much better: "Ma cousine se porte mieux, mais, pour que je sois contente, il faut que ce soit tout à fait bien et je ne me déciderai à retourner à Paris que quand j'aurai atteint ce but-là; elle se trouve à merveille ici, rien ne le prouve mieux que son désir d'y rester, quoique sa Mathilde ne soit pas avec elle" ["My cousin is doing better, but for me to be happy, she needs to be completely healthy and I will decide to return to Paris only when I have attained that goal; she is so happy here, nothing proves this more than her wish to remain, even though Mathilde is not with her"] (*UO*, 185). In a letter to another friend, Mélanie Lemarcis, Cottin described why spending the winter (1803–4) in Bagnères seemed a logical choice: "Voici les avantages: une grande économie, chose très nécessaire après un long et dispendieux voyage; une température plus douce qu'à Toulouse; un excellent maître de dessin; beaucoup de ressources pour la musique; des bains salutaires tout l'hiver; des eaux restaurantes qui font du bien dans toutes les saisons; une grande solitude où nous pourrions nous occuper de nos enfants et où je pourrais travailler à mon aise" ["Here are the advantages: considerable savings, something very necessary after a long and costly trip; a milder climate than in Toulouse; an excellent drawing teacher; many resources for music instruction; beneficial baths all winter long; rejuvenating water that does one good all year round; total isolation where we can take care of our children and where I can work at my leisure"] (*MC*, 358). Cottin felt that Julie's health could be put at risk if they left too soon: "Je vous avoue que la santé de Julie est un des grands motifs qui me font craindre le séjour de Paris. Un hiver doux lui serait si bon; quel dommage de gâter le bien qu'elle a gagné!" ["I confess to you that Julie's health is one of the main reasons I fear living in Paris. A mild winter would do her so much good; how sad it would be to lose the benefits she has gained!"] (359).

The benefits were not all Julie's: the "restoring" waters of Bagnères had worked their wonder on Cottin as well. The restoration of her health she described in the letter cited earlier (see chapter 2) referred specifically to the return of menstruation, something she considered nothing short of miraculous. Why menstruation resumed during the trip to Bagnères is unclear. Cottin attributed it directly to the air, the water, and the baths of Bagnères, and perhaps she was right. It is possible that the change in altitude, the bath treatments in the spa, and distance from the pressures of Paris, family, and society all contributed to this return to normalcy. Whatever the cause, the effect on Cottin was dramatic: "comme mon coeur a palpité de joie dans ces temps-là" ["how my heart leapt with joy in those days!"].[1] Cottin had made the trip to Bagnères at a time of increasing religious devotion in her life. She read the restoration as a sign that God had led her to Bagnères to heal her, to make her whole once again in preparation for a greater destiny than she had ever known. For her to connect the pilgrimage, the act of faith, with the reward of potential maternity seems entirely logical, given her state of mind. Cottin herself was convinced that it was evidence of the hand of God in her life, signaling her election as a vessel worthy at last to bear children.

In Bagnères she claimed to have been reborn "à une vie nouvelle" ["to a new life"] (*UO*, 218).

This explains why she would look upon her introduction to Hyacinthe Azaïs as more than coincidence. She thought that if God had brought her there to make her whole, it was for a reason. "Cet accident . . . a duré presque continuellement jusqu'à mon voyage à Bagnères," she wrote to Azaïs. "Lorsqu'il cessa, je crus que Dieu même me montrait qu'il m'avait amenée là pour être à vous"["This condition . . . persisted almost continually until my trip to Bagnères. When it ceased, I believed that God himself was showing me that he had led me there to be yours"].[2] The return of menstruation changed the way Cottin viewed herself; she could now look upon herself as complete, whole, and acceptable. For the first time since being widowed, she could allow herself to entertain ideas of marriage and family.

Evidently her relationship with the thirty-seven-year-old Azaïs had at first been strictly platonic, founded on intellectual compatibility. But with the return of menstruation, Cottin let herself believe marriage was possible. The self-made theologian and philosopher had begun to exercise a great influence over Cottin's life and thought. His past had much of the romantic in it: he had, for instance, been a monk at one time, only to be released from his vows later at his own request. He, like Cottin, had also been ordered by revolutionary officials to leave the country but had chosen concealment instead, spending eighteen months hidden away in an attic, during which he had plenty of time to think, read, and write. The result was a rather peculiar system of theophilosophy that he hoped would make him famous. At first, Azaïs refused to reveal his system to Cottin, fearing, he said, that she might accidentally talk of it to others and rob him of the fame he hoped to win when he unveiled it in his book. When he did finally acquiesce to her request, Cottin admitted to being left rather disappointed, apparently because the system relied heavily on logic. Her approach to religion was very close to that of Chateaubriand: "j'étais née pour les religions de foi et d'amour, et non pour celles de clarté et de raison" ["I was born for religions of faith and love, not for those based on clarity and reason"] (*UO*, 204). Azaïs's approach therefore ran counter to her own, and she confessed: "là où il n'y a pas de mystères incompréhensibles, il me manque quelque chose" ["where there are no incomprehensible mysteries, something is missing for me"] (*MC*, 58). She resisted any intellectual system that, while attempting to provide the same moral values and spiritual reassurance as Christianity, eliminated reliance on revealed religion: "je ne me verrais arracher qu'avec douleur mes pensées chrétiennes; soit qu'elles tiennent ou non à des préjugés, je les chéris et je voudrais vivre et mourir avec elles. Je les défends avec obstination contre cette nouvelle lumière qui me montre bien le même résultat, mais qui ne m'y conduit pas par le même chemin, et c'est ce chemin qui m'était doux et que je regretterais lors même qu'on en enseignerait un meilleur" ["Throwing away my Christian beliefs would only cause me pain; whether or not they are based on personal bias, I treasure them and want to live and die with them. I defend them obstinately against this new light which shows me the same result but which doesn't take me down the same path to get there, a path I have found comforting and that I would miss even if someone showed me a better one"] (*UO*, 195–96).

This professed resistance to Azaïs's philosophy, however, gradually weakened under the influence of his eloquence, and Cottin became a true convert of the man she liked to call "le solitaire des Pyrénées" ["the hermit of the Pyrenees"] (*UO*, 210). She found it impossible to resist talking or writing about him to everyone in her entourage, often in the most extravagant of hyperboles and always to their annoyance. Julie and others simply could not understand her attraction to the philosopher, but for Cottin the magnetism was real and irresistible. Azaïs's system had a beneficial effect on her life, Cottin thought, because it helped her see she had been heading down the wrong road before her arrival in Bagnères; in Paris, she had been consumed by *coquetterie,* as she called it, and needed to be brought up short. "Il m'a montré le journal de sa vie," she wrote. "Oh! quel trésor d'instruction qu'une pareille lecture! Après l'avoir lu, tout a été dit. J'ai senti que je ne ferais plus une faute grave dans ma vie, et que la passion n'aurait plus de prise sur mon âme. Je suis donc dans un état doux, paisible, heureux" ["He showed me his diary. Oh! What instructive reading it was! After reading it, there was nothing left to be said. I felt I would never commit another serious mistake in my life and that passion would no longer have any hold on me. I am, as a result, in a calm, peaceful, and happy state of mind"] (*MC*, 359).

Cottin became more and more convinced that she had been led to Bagnères for a reason: "Je ne sais quelle Providence m'a amenée au fond des Pyrénées, m'y a fait passer un hiver entier dans la plus profonde solitude, mais assurément il y a du ciel dans cette Providence-là. . . . [N]on, je ne pourrais vous dépeindre l'état intérieur où je me trouve, l'expression en passe mes moyens et je ne puis que répéter: *je suis heureuse"* ["I don't know what destiny brought me to the heart of the Pyrenees and caused me to spend an entire winter in the deepest solitude, but assuredly there is something divine in that destiny. . . . [N]o, I couldn't describe for you the state I am in, I don't have the words to describe it, and all I can do is keep repeating: *I am happy*"] (*UO*, 217). Writing to Madame de Pastoret, she claimed: "Sans doute la Providence m'a envoyée auprès de lui [Azaïs], au moment où j'étais le plus disposée à l'entendre, et peut-être dois-je autant de reconnaissance à la Providence qu'à lui; aussi j'aime à les confondre ensemble, à recevoir leurs bienfaits comme venant également du ciel et à les réunir dans mon coeur pour les aimer de la même tendresse"] ["Without doubt God sent me here to [Azaïs] at a time when I was most prepared to listen to him, and perhaps I owe as much to God as I do to him; and so I like to consider them as one, to accept both blessings as if they came from heaven and to unite them in my heart in order to love them both with the same tenderness"] (231). God had restored her fertility, the most precious of all gifts he could give, and now Azaïs offered the possibility of marriage and family. It was indeed as if a whole new life were opening up before her: "maintenant je renais pour ainsi dire avec le printemps à une vie nouvelle où je ne vois que bienfait et jouissance autour de moi" ["I am now being reborn, so to speak, with springtime itself into a new life where I see only goodness and happiness surrounding me"] (218). "En vérité, madame," she exclaimed, "je serais presque tentée de croire que c'est ici le pays des miracles" ["Truly, I am almost tempted to believe that this is the land of miracles"] (221).

In May 1804, Julie left Bagnères for Toulouse to take care of some family business. Ten days later, Cottin herself left Bagnères, accompanied by a M. de Cardaillac, a friend of hers, who took her to his château in Lomné (on the road to Toulouse); Cottin stayed there for a short while, chaperoned by the mother and sisters of her host. She waited for Julie at Lomné, then returned with her to Bagnères to spend a few more weeks. On 16 July 1804, Cottin obtained a passport from city officials to travel to Barèges. From there, she traveled to Tonneins, arriving by 22 August, and she was back in Champlan shortly thereafter (*MC*, 60).

The hope of future happiness endured after her return to Champlan, and to Azaïs, who had stayed behind in Bagnères, she described this new "fullness" she was experiencing: "Tous les enthousiasmes sont revenus se placer dans mon coeur. Est-ce votre amour qui les a produits? Est-ce à vous que je dois cette plénitude de vie qui quelquefois m'oppresse jusqu'à crier, jusqu'à mourir? Comment vous expliquer ces instants où mon coeur se gonfle d'une joie dont il ignore la cause, mais qui mêle quelque chose de divin à tous les sentiments qu'il éprouve? . . . Je suis à vous comme le monde est à Dieu, je suis votre ouvrage et votre propriété" ["A zest for life has returned to my heart. Has your love produced it? Is it to you that I owe this fullness of life that sometimes overcomes me so much that I want to cry out and even die? How can I describe these moments when my heart swells with a joy of unknown origin but which blends something of the divine with all the emotions it feels? . . . I am yours like the world is God's, you have created me and I belong to you"] (*MC*, 363).

But, as we noted earlier, Cottin soon relapsed into her former amenorrheic condition. Knowing that for Azaïs the creation of children was the only viable condition for marriage, she felt compelled to write and tell him the crushing truth about her infertility. Evidently, God had not meant her to know the kind of plenitude she had envisioned for herself. Since fullness or plenitude was God's affair in the first place, then perhaps he meant her to discover a different dimension to the word and a different answer to the question of her defectiveness: "Déjà depuis longtemps, je tourne mon coeur vers Dieu; sans doute la seule amitié y laisserait du vide, mais Dieu pourra peut-être le remplir; et vous, mon ami, n'y resterez-vous pas aussi?" ["For a long time now, I have been reaching out to God; friendship alone will certainly not fill the emptiness in my heart, but perhaps God will be able to fill it; and you, my friend, will you not also be there?"].[3] She concluded her letter with the thought that perhaps a return to Bagnères would work the same magic but acknowledged that her age would likely preclude any such hope: "Mais de pareils calculs, de telles attentes ne sont permises qu'à la jeunesse [*sic*]: ma jeunesse est passée. Ah! mon ami, si je la pleure, ce n'est que du regret de ne pouvoir vous la donner" ["Only the young can undertake those kinds of projects, make such attempts; my youth has passed. Oh, my friend, if I weep at its passing, it is only because I regret not being able to give it to you"].[4]

Cottin knew that the revelation of her infertility would be fatal to her relationship with Azaïs; indeed, he seems to have been little touched by Cottin's confession, seeing it rather as his own misfortune to have been attracted to a woman incapable of being a mother. Trying to give closure to this sad episode in her life, Cottin wrote him: "Adieu mon ami: mon sage et vertueux ami, mon bienfaiteur et mon guide, cessons de nous voir mais ne cessons pas de nous estimer, je n'ose dire plus. Cependant, pourquoi oublierions-nous un amour dont l'innocence n'eut point à rougir, un amour pur, irréprochable, fondé sur les plus nobles motifs et auquel nous devons peut-être plusieurs de nos vertus?" ["Goodbye, my friend, my wise and virtuous friend, my benefactor and my guide, let us cease to see one another but let us not cease to admire one another, I dare not say anything more. Yet, why forget an innocent love that had nothing to be ashamed of, a pure love, exemplary, founded on the noblest of motives and to which we perhaps owe many of our virtues?"] (*UO*, 270). She described her final state of mind to Azaïs: "Je suis bien, j'ai vaincu l'orage, le calme a succédé; j'ai dans l'âme une résignation douce, tendre, entière. Je crois que ce que Dieu a décidé est le mieux possible; puisque ni vous ni moi n'avons la force de lever l'obstacle qu'il a mis entre nous, apparemment qu'il nous est bon qu'un obstacle nous sépare" ["I am well, I have conquered the storm, calm has followed; sweet, tender, and complete resignation fills my soul. I believe that what God has decided is for the best; because neither you nor I have the power to remove the barrier he has placed between us, it is apparently for our benefit that a barrier separate us"] (272). With this declaration, Cottin pronounced an end to the emotional relationship that had dominated two of the most turbulent years of her life; in much the same way as Mathilde, the heroine she created during this experience, she buried her love and remained "sans liens" ["without ties"] (1:398).

Upon her return to the Paris area in August of 1804, Cottin had contacted her new editor, Joseph Michaud, about the possibilities of publishing her recently completed *Mathilde*. Michaud, one of the founders of the famous *Dictionnaire biographique*, had gained notoriety writing a history of the Crusades (*MC*, 61). During the Revolution, he had favored the royalists, a position that had kept him on the run when he was not actually in prison. Michaud had finally decided to get out of politics and, with his brother and another fellow named Giguet, had founded a press. Cottin met Michaud before her trip to the Pyrenees, and he had visited her at Champlan; during her sojourn in Bagnères, he wrote to her several times, discussing for the most part simply literary matters.

Upon her return to Paris, Michaud's interest in Cottin evidently developed into something beyond a simple business relationship. This was perhaps once more the consequence of Cottin's habit of confiding in people and the intensity of her emotional attachment in friendship. Michaud evidently mistook her friendship for romantic interest and began to write her about the feelings he was beginning to have for her. Cottin was vexed that she had allowed him to assume things she did not feel from her side, especially since she was still involved so deeply with Azaïs at the time. She insisted that their relationship remain at the friendship level. In his reply, Michaud admitted: "Vous m'avez défendu de trop vous aimer; je vous aime davantage, beaucoup plus que je vous aimais. Cependant j'ai fait tout ce que vous désiriez, je suis tel que vous l'avez voulu" ["You have forbidden me to love you too much; I love you more, far more than I loved you before. Nevertheless, I have done what you wanted, I am as you wished"] (*MC*, 372). He did his best to reassure her that he would take care to keep his feelings within the bounds she had set: "Il n'y a rien de dangereux ni pour vous ni pour moi dans mon affection. Elle n'est point le produit de l'exaltation ni de l'enthousiasme, elle n'est point née subitement et à l'improviste. Je vous aime beaucoup, autant que j'ai jamais aimé, mais je vous aime comme on aime la campagne, comme on aime la bonté ou la vertu avec tous ses charmes. . . . Je ne parlerai que le langage que vous voudrez; je ne vous demanderai rien en échange de mes sentiments, je me contenterai de votre amitié" ["There is nothing dangerous either for you or for myself in my affection. It is not the result of rapture or enthusiasm, it was not born suddenly or unexpectedly. I love you very much, as much as I have ever loved, but I love you as one loves the countryside, as one loves goodness or virtue with all its charms. . . . I will speak only the language that you wish; I will ask nothing of you in exchange for my feelings, I will be satisfied with your friendship"] (374).

Although Michaud was to be the editor of her new novel, other publishers were interested. Dentu, for instance, wanted to buy the manuscript and made inquiries about the possibility through Cottin's brother-in-law André. Though Cottin felt obligated to Michaud because of her earlier commitment to him, she nevertheless gave proof of a developing business sense by asking André to find out what Dentu would be willing to pay: "Dans cet embarras, je n'écrirai point à ce libraire passionné [Dentu], mais je voudrais bien qu'indirectement vous puissiez savoir de lui ce qu'il offrirait pour l'objet de sa passion [le manuscrit de *Mathilde*], parce que ce serait une base sur laquelle on pourrait traiter avec M. Michaud" ["In this difficult situation, I won't write to that eager bookseller [Dentu], but I would appreciate it if indirectly you could find out from him what he would offer for the object of his passion [the *Mathilde* manuscript], because it would be useful in dealing with M. Michaud"] (*MC*, 374). In the end, Cottin signed a contract with Michaud for 7,000 francs, giving him the rights to publish the first edition of *Mathilde* as well as new editions of her earlier novels.

When *Mathilde* appeared in August 1805, it quickly captured the reading public's attention. One of Cottin's biographers, Arnelle, comments: "Ce livre a eu un succès colossal; l'imagerie populaire s'en est emparé; on en a fait des sujets de pendule, des décorations de vases empires, en un mot, une vulgarisation flatteuse, comme pour les tableaux qu'on représente actuellement sur des tapis, ces orgues de barbarie de la peinture" ["The book was a colossal success; its subject matter was picked up by commercial artists and used to decorate clocks and Empire-style vases, in a word, a flattering vulgarization, like the paintings we see reproduced on rugs nowadays, those street organs of painting"] (*UO*, 326). Perhaps a more reliable indication of the novel's success, however, was Ledentu's decision in 1844, when publishing an edition of Cottin's *Oeuvres complètes*, to place *Mathilde* as the opening novel—followed by *Claire d'Albe* and *Elisabeth*—in the first volume of a two-volume set. Knowing that buyers are unlikely to purchase only one volume of a published set of works, Ledentu included Cottin's best-sellers in the first volume, thereby virtually assuring the sale of the second volume as well. This strategy appears to have been common practice among early-nineteenth-century publishing houses. When Ladvocat, for example, began publication of Chateaubriand's *Oeuvres complètes* in 1826—a collection that would ultimately total twenty-eight volumes—he started in the middle, with the first volume issued numbered as volume 16. It included *Atala* and *René*, by far the most popular of Chateaubriand's works. Those who bought volume 16 were thereby committed to the ultimate purchase over the next five years of all remaining twenty-seven volumes in Ladvocat's series.

Mathilde; ou, Mémoires tirés de l'histoire des croisades is noteworthy in many ways. First, it is the longest of Cottin's novels; the Michaud edition of August 1805 was a six-volume set. Because of Cottin's tendency to work on two or three novels simultaneously, it took her nearly six years to complete *Mathilde*, qualifying it as her most extended writing project by far. Second, it was her first nonepistolary novel, written from a narrative stance of zero focalization rather than from internal as was her style in the earlier novels. Third, it was the first novel published with her name openly displayed as the author; all three earlier novels—*Claire d'Albe*, *Malvina*, and *Amélie Mansfield*—had been published anonymously. This may be a significant fact; from the outset, Cottin publicly declared her ownership of the characters and ideas found in *Mathilde*. Obviously, she felt no embarrassment, no need to hide behind anonymity, in telling this story that she considered a defense of the Christian faith's ability to bridle human passions and by so doing to bring happiness. At least, on the surface, that is what the story seemed to say.

In this novel, Cottin sets up many opposing forces, the most important of which is the tension between two women: Mathilde, the sixteen-year-old sister of Richard the Lionheart, an "innocente colombe" ["innocent dove"] (1:9) destined for the convent, and Agnès, the princess of Jerusalem who denies the Christian faith because of her love for an infidel and who takes up arms against her own people and religious heritage. These two confront one another at pivotal points in the narrative and their ultimate destinies provide much of the novel's moralistic tone.

The novel begins with Pope Gregory VIII preaching a new crusade to recover Jerusalem, which has fallen to the Saracen king Saladin. Richard I, king of England, and Philippe-Auguste, the French monarch, agree to march at the head of the assembled Christian armies, but before embarking for Palestine, Richard goes back to London to invest his brother John. He arranges with his fiancée, Bérengère, to meet him in Sicily, where they will be married. Before Richard leaves England, he expresses a desire to witness the ceremony in which his youngest sister, Mathilde, will take her vows to begin her life as a nun. Mathilde, sixteen years old, has been raised in a cloister with the purest of companions; she lives in "innocence parfaite" ["perfect innocence"], the narrative informs us, ignorant equally of the existence of evil and the merits of virtue (1:7). Knowing of the world and its dangers only through the abbess's descriptions, Mathilde anticipates the day of her vows with joy.

As king, Richard, accompanied by Guillaume, the archbishop of Tyre, is allowed to enter areas of the cloister where no man has ever set foot. In talking with Mathilde, the two men describe the Holy Land, the suffering of the Christians there, and the loss of the holy sites to the Saracens, all of which causes Mathilde to express the desire to "take up the cross" with her brother and visit the Holy Land before separating herself from the world. Her request is granted enthusiastically; she prepares to leave the convent, dressed in the brilliant white habit of the novice, on which the abbess places a shining cross. The abbess says to the archbishop: "ce n'est point la princesse d'Angleterre que je vous recommande, mais la future épouse de Dieu; c'est le plus beau de tous les titres, sans doute" ["This is not the princess of England that I am giving you, but the future bride of God; of all titles, that is, without doubt, the most beautiful"] (1:8). She warns Mathilde to give no ear to the enchanting voices of the world and to concentrate on her celestial spouse. Mathilde is now poised at the brink of entering the world for the first time in her life; her look of fright causes the abbess to give her a reliquary containing a piece of the true cross, which the abbess has always worn. She tells Mathilde to press it to her breast whenever she is tempted and it will save her.

The world seems very large and menacing to Mathilde; the sea voyage and the language of the warriors and sailors are in striking contrast with the life of the cloister she has known. Upon arrival at Messina, she meets Bérengère and the two become fast friends instantly. Problems between Philippe and Richard make Richard delay his marriage; not until he conquers Cyprus will he marry Bérengère. When Guy de Lusignan, king of Jerusalem, hears of Richard's conquest of Cyprus, he comes to see him. Lusignan reveals that he is being challenged for his right to rule by Conrad, marquis de Montferrat and ruler of Tyre; Philippe-Auguste has declared in favor of Conrad, and now Lusignan comes to Richard to seek his support. Tyre, the only city controlled by the Christians, has closed its gates to Lusignan and declared itself in revolt. Richard, jealous of Philippe, is only too happy to have this opportunity to oppose him; Lusignan and Richard swear mutual allegiance and become friends.

Mathilde attends her future sister-in-law at the magnificent wedding; although he is a married man, Lusignan falls in love with Mathilde at first sight. Only a few days after his wedding, Richard is anxious to get on with his crusade. Lusignan warns him the seas are covered with enemy vessels and that Malek Adhel, the brother of Saladin and the most feared warrior in Asia, commands them and has sworn death to all the kings of Europe. Richard does not want his new wife and Mathilde to risk these dangers and thus decides to have them follow later in a separate ship, after he has reached Ptolemais. Outnumbered, Richard nevertheless fights his way through the enemy fleet and arrives victorious at Ptolemais.

Upon his arrival at Ptolemais with Richard, Lusignan learns that his wife, Sibylle, has died. Lusignan had become king of Jerusalem through his marriage to Sibylle, daughter of Baudouin; with her now gone, the right to the throne will pass to the younger sister, Isabelle, who is married to Conrad. Lusignan insists on his continued right to the kingship but is not supported in this by Philippe-Auguste and the troops he commands. The crusaders' camp is consequently divided into different loyalties. Conrad refuses to help the crusaders with their seige of Ptolemais until Richard accepts him as king of Jerusalem. Dissension almost brings the Christians to war among themselves.

Richard sends for Bérengère and Mathilde and waits impatiently for their arrival. Mathilde, from her side, is shocked at the openly stated passion of her sister-in-law for her new husband: "étonnée d'un langage si nouveau, [Mathilde] s'alarmait de l'entendre, et se croyait coupable de prêter l'oreille aux accents d'un pur et légitime amour" ["astonished by a language new to her, [Mathilde] grew alarmed at hearing it and considered herself guilty for having listened to feelings springing from a pure and legitimate love"] (1:16). She tells the archbishop her troubles and he begins to view her as "l'Eve céleste au premier réveil du monde" ["the heavenly Eve when the world was new"] (1:16). He believes her to be a saint: "courageuse et modeste, la jeune vierge dédaignait tous les terrestres biens, et traversait le monde, occupée seulement du ciel" ["courageous and unassuming, the young virgin held all earthly things in contempt and traveled through life with her eyes focused on heaven alone"] (1:17).

Their boat is blown off course and beached; the Saracens arrive and give battle but are about to lose when Malek Adhel appears. The archbishop is sure they are doomed but, after defeating the crew handily, Malek Adhel promises Bérengère safety in his palace and tells her that her entourage will not be enslaved as long as they swear not to try joining up with the camp of the crusaders until Saladin has had a chance to negotiate a ransom with Richard for his new queen. The queen is satisfied with this but asks that she not be separated from Mathilde. When Malek Adhel sees Mathilde's face in the daylight, he is overcome by her beauty. He has her taken to his ship, where he tries to hold her hand and talk to her; she is horrified by his advances and falls at the feet of the archbishop, who then tries to explain to Malek Adhel that this girl has taken vows of chastity: "l'approche d'un homme est pour elle une souillure, et jusqu'à ce jour, nul chevalier chrétien n'a osé regarder d'un oeil profane la vierge du Seigneur" ["she feels defiled by the presence of a man, and until today, no Christian knight has dared look upon the Lord's virgin in a worldly way"] (1:20). Malek Adhel criticizes Christianity: "j'y vois les effets de cette religion fanatique que vous nommez la *très sainte*, tandis que vous taxez la nôtre d'être impie et barbare; cependant, toute barbare qu'elle est, jamais elle n'a commandé à nos guerriers d'aller ravager votre patrie, ni à de jeunes et célestes beautés de quitter le monde et ses plaisirs pour s'ensevelir toutes vivantes dans un tombeau" ["I see in this the effects of that fanatical religion that you call the *most holy one*, whereas you accuse ours of being ungodly and barbaric; nevertheless, as barbaric as ours is, never has it ordered its warriors to ravage your lands or asked its young, heavenly beauties to leave the world and its pleasures behind in order to bury themselves alive in a tomb"] (1:21). But Malek respects Mathilde's vows; she is allowed to live in his palace at Damiette, along with the queen and the archbishop. For her part, Mathilde is surprised to realize that she has not seen the marks of Satan in Malek Adhel as she had been led to believe she would.

The Christians are placed in a palace near Malek's main palace and are allowed to worship and visit together as they please. The gardens around their palace, though adjoining those of the harem, are separated by high walls with no communication between them. One day, while walking in the garden, Mathilde and Bérengère are surprised to find a slave girl who tells them: "je suis une malheureuse souillée du plus noir des crimes; j'ai renié mon Dieu et ma patrie, pour suivre en ce lieu impie ma royale et coupable maîtresse" ["I am an unfortunate woman defiled by the blackest of crimes; I have denied my God and my country in order to follow my royal and guilty mistress to this place"] (1:37). The slave girl explains that her mistress, Agnès, the princess of Jerusalem and a Christian, has fallen in love with Malek Adhel and given herself to him. Agnès has followed Malek to his palace where, now despised by him, she is treated like all the other slaves. According to the slave girl, Malek had recently announced to all his women that he was going to give them away; she claims that Malek had changed because of a "pure love" he had found, similar to that which Christian knights feel. Agnès has told him she wants simply to leave but he will not let her, and she appears to be dying of shame and grief. Bérengère understands immediately that Mathilde is the source of the pure love mentioned as motive for Malek's strange behavior, but Mathilde has no idea of her possible connection to the situation.

The passion that had led Agnès into treachery and enslavement bears a striking similarity to that driving the behavior of other Cottin heroines such as Claire and Amélie: "Aussi le sentiment que lui inspire Malek Adhel ne fut point cette tendresse que la

5: *MATHILDE* AND THE MIRACLE OF BAGNÈRES

vertu permet aux femmes: ce fut une de ces passions effrénées, telle qu'il en naît dans le coeur des guerriers, et qui, semblables à un torrent enflammé, se répandent à flots précipités, sans craindre ni l'éclat ni le bruit. Ah! que ne doit-on pas attendre d'une vierge qui a rompu une fois les chaînes de l'austère pudeur! elle tombe avec d'autant plus de force que ses liens étaient plus étroits" ["The feeling Malek Adhel inspired in her was not the tenderness that virtue allows women to have: it was one of those unbridled passions such as is born in the hearts of warriors and that, like a raging flood, spreads with rushing waves, without fear of scandal or rumor. Ah! what can one expect from a virgin once she has broken the bonds of strict chastity! The more restrictive her life as a virgin, the greater her fall"] (1:43). Because this description of confinement resembles Mathilde's own situation, the reader is led to wonder what fate awaits her.

At this point in the narrative, Agnès herself appears at the entrance to the grove; she is angry at Mathilde for having stolen the heart of the one she loves. Mathilde takes pity on Agnès and invites her to sleep in her bedroom that night. In the middle of the night, Mathilde is awakened by a horrible scream. She runs to Agnès, who then tells her what it is like to have given everything up for passion:

Tu frémis, Mathilde, et jamais tes oreilles n'ouïrent de pareils forfaits. Eh bien! tu ne sais pas tout encore; non, tu ne sais pas jusqu'à quel excès d'impiété l'amour a pu m'entraîner. J'ai désiré l'anéantissement de l'empire du Christ, parce qu'il peut s'élever contre celui de mon amant; j'ai désiré voir cet amant régner seul sur tous les rois et les mondes enchaînés; j'allais le suivre à l'armée, combattre contre la cause que je soutenais autrefois, et, pour défendre une tête adorée, lever l'épée contre mon propre sang et le Dieu de mes pères.... Enfin, dans ce moment même, quand Guillaume [l'archevêque] m'ouvre la voie du repentir, et que mon ingrat époux m'abandonne et me hait, l'idée de le fuir, de m'en séparer à jamais, est plus terrible à mes yeux que celle de ma damnation éternelle.

[You tremble, Mathilde, and never before have your ears heard such crimes. Well, you don't know everything yet; no, you don't know to what excesses of impiety love has led me. I have wished for the annihilation of Christ's kingdom, because it could rise up against that of my lover; I wanted to see that lover reign supreme among kings over all the enslaved world; I was going to follow him into the army, fight against the cause I had formerly upheld, and, in order to defend my lover, raise the sword against my own blood and the God of my fathers.... Indeed, even now, as Guillaume [the archbishop] opens the road of repentance to me, and my ingrate of a husband abandons me and hates me, the thought of leaving him, of separating from him forever, is more horrible in my eyes than eternal damnation."] (1:50)

This declaration of female rebellion echoes passages in Cottin's earlier novels; Claire d'Albe and Amélie Mansfield both make similar statements. In this case, however, the main female character, Mathilde, does not make the statement but is shown reacting to it—the rebellious discourse is relocated to a separate and isolated voice outside the center of the narrative. Mathilde, the innocent virgin, is shocked into silence by the blasphemy she hears: "Pendant tout ce discours, Mathilde était demeurée immobile et tremblante: l'expression d'une passion aussi effréné lui faisait horreur: incapable de répondre un seul mot à des discours si nouveaux pour elle, impatiente de s'affranchir de la honte de les écouter, elle ne pouvait se résoudre pourtant à laisser Agnès seule en proie à son affreux délire" ["During this speech, Mathilde had remained motionless and trembling: the expression of such an unbridled passion horrified her: incapable of answering a single word to speech that was so new to her, impatient to free herself from the shame of listening to it, she nevertheless could not bring herself to abandon Agnès while possessed by her dreadful delirium"] (1:51). Finding the archbishop, Mathilde tells him: "Mon père, la princesse de Jérusalem est fort mal, je ne sais quelle fièvre l'agite; mais sa raison est entièrement perdue, car elle ne parle que des ravissements du crime, des délices de l'impiété, et Malek Adhel lui semble préférable à Dieu même" ["My father, the princess of Jerusalem is very sick, I don't know what fever has seized her; but she has lost her reason entirely; for she speaks only of the pleasures of crime, of the delights of ungodliness, and she seems to prefer Malek Adhel over God himself"] (1:51). Guillaume stops her in mid-sentence, telling her that a pure mouth should not be caught repeating such things.

This is but the first of several confrontations Cottin creates between the innocent virgin and the rebellious woman-warrior of her novel. She relishes the bipolar relationship of this pair of women; it is as if she has made her previous characters confront one another now in a final showdown, to see who will come out victorious. The irony is that Cottin as author controls the outcome and yet she will prolong the final resolution of the struggle until the very last moment. Nothing is decided quickly in this novel; every conflict must be drawn out to excruciating lengths.

Mathilde's commitment to the Christian God and her moral code will be tested in every conceivable way until, tried by the fire of passion, she comes out the victor.

Wanting to get a big ransom out of Richard, Saladin will not allow Malek to return Bérengère to her husband and commands that the captive be transferred to Cairo. Mathilde, who is to be released, devises a ruse in which she substitutes herself for Bérengère. During the voyage, Malek makes a confession of his love for Mathilde to the woman he believes is the queen. When Mathilde reveals her true identity, he tells her there is no other who could love her more powerfully than he. Mathilde cannot help but believe him, but the narrator adds: "Qu'il y a de dangers dans cette pensée! et qu'il est difficile au coeur le plus humble, le plus pur, de se défendre d'un tendre orgueil à l'idée d'être l'objet d'une passion profonde, unique, telle que jamais nul homme sur terre n'en connut de semblable!" ["What dangers there are in that thought! and how difficult it is for the humblest and purest heart to defend itself against the vanity of being the object of a deep passion, a unique passion, a passion that no man on earth has ever known!"] (1:118). Continuing with this moralizing tone, the narrator comments:

> Ainsi Mathilde, satisfaite de se conserver chaste, va donc oublier de se conserver pure, et pourvu que sa vertu demeure inébranlable, elle ne songera plus que ces entrevues avec un homme, ces discours passionnés qu'elle écoute, sont autant d'atteintees à son innocence; que ces mêmes choses, qu'elle veut regarder comme peu importantes aujourd'hui, lui eussent paru criminelles à son arrivée à Damiette; elle ne songera point que c'est ainsi qu'en négligeant de compter tous les pas qu'on fait dans la carrière de la séduction, et que se rassurant sur tous ceux qu'on fait encore, par la certitude de ne pas aller plus avant, on est entraîné par une pente insensible jusqu'au fond de ce gouffre des passions humaines, où il n'y a de choix qu'entre la mort et la honte.

> [Thus Mathilde, satisfied with preserving her chastity, will forget to preserve her purity, and as long as her virtue remains unshaken, she will no longer imagine that these meetings with a man, these passionate speeches she hears, are just so many attacks on her innocence; that these same things, which she wants to consider as being of little importance today, would have appeared sinful to her when she first arrived in Damiette; she will not imagine that it is in neglecting to count every step one takes along the path of seduction, and in reassuring oneself about all the steps that one is still taking, that a person is led down an imperceptible slope into the depths of the abyss of

human passions, where the only choice left is between death and shame.] (1:118)

Cottin's choice of zero focalization in *Mathilde* gives this kind of speech an authority not felt in her earlier texts; when characters in an epistolary novel, for instance, give themselves over to moralizing, the reader is allowed greater freedom in accepting or rejecting the claims. In zero focalization, however, the narrative voice assumes the role of the omniscient creator; the author speaks as or for God. And the narrator's final statement in this section sounds very much like a pronouncement from heaven: "ce n'est pas en obéissant à ses passions, c'est en leur résistant qu'on se procure la vraie paix du coeur" ["it is not in succumbing to one's passions, it is in resisting them that one gains true peace of mind"] (1:118). To prove this, Cottin shows Mathilde trying to study the Bible to help her forget her growing love, but she cannot maintain her concentration. Mathilde vows that she will not be overtaken by emotion, but the narrator wonders: "Ô chaste vierge! qu'es-tu devenue? Se peut-il que l'ennemi ait vaincu ton courage? et cet amour contre lequel tu te débats, s'est-il accru à un tel point que tu ne trouves déjà plus dans ta modestie assez de voiles pour te le cacher?" ["O chaste virgin! what have you become? Is it possible that the enemy has overcome your courage? And this love against which you struggle, has it already grown to the point where your modesty no longer has enough veils to hide it from you?"] (1:119).

Agnès, from her side, has already discovered the trickery and vows she will kill Mathilde. Clothed in men's armor and wielding a sword, she crashes into Mathilde's room; Malek throws himself in the way and takes the blow. Mathilde, thinking Malek is going to die, faints. Malek tries to seize Agnès but she holds him off with the sword and says something, which allows him to realize who it is under the armor. Agnès then runs away with Malek in pursuit.

As readers, we are allowed to see every vacillation in Mathilde's soul; each time she vows to do something, her heart pulls her in another direction. She battles constantly to free herself of love's attraction, sinning in her desires and then immediately repenting and punishing herself for allowing herself to stray: "Hélas! où sont les tranquilles plaisirs, les paisibles joies de son adolescence? qu'a-t-elle gagné à chercher d'autres biens, et qu'a-t-elle rencontré hors de sa retraite? d'épaisses ténèbres, de cruelles agitations, et une infinité de maux dont les noms lui étaient même inconnus dans son premier état d'innocence" ["Alas! where are the simple pleasures, the bliss of her adolescence? What has she gained in seeking other riches, and what has she encountered outside her sanctuary? Darkness, cruel agitation, and an infinite number of troubles unknown to her in her original state of innocence"] (1:138). Indeed, like the Eve she had been compared to earlier in the text, Mathilde feels her innocence now compromised by the temptation of strong desires, and she decides to flee into the desert. She begs Malek to allow her to make a pilgrimage to a ruin in the Egyptian desert, home of a famous holy man. This flight into the desert will retrace the very path taken by the only mortal woman capable of resisting all passion, the Virgin herself. Mathilde rejoices in the thought that her suffering in the desert will not only expiate her sins but, more importantly, penetrate deep enough into her heart to destroy her forbidden love.

After three days in the desert, Mathilde and her group arrive at the shores of the Red Sea; from there, she is able to lead them directly to the saint's abode. Even here, with the hermit's example before her eyes, Mathilde still finds herself combating her desires:

> Tout en larmes, elle offre mille fois son coeur à Dieu, s'efforce de laisser le passé dans l'oubli, l'avenir à la Providence, et de donner le présent au ciel; mais toujours un invincible penchant l'entraîne vers d'autres intérêts que les siens, le nom de Malek Adhel se mêle à toutes ses prières; si elle les commence pour elle, c'est pour lui qu'elle les finit; et quand elle demande à Dieu ses grâces victorieuses, dans lesquelles il n'entre pas moins de puissance que d'amour, et que son beau visage se colore d'un feu plus vif, ce n'est pas alors pour elle qu'elle prie.

> [In tears, she offers her heart to God a thousand times, tries to leave the past behind her, the future to Providence, and give the present to heaven; but an invincible attraction always draws her toward interests other than her own, the name of Malek Adhel enters into all her prayers; if she begins praying for herself, she finishes praying for him; and when she asks God for his grace, as powerful as love, and her beautiful face brightens, it is not for herself that she is praying.] (1:149)

Her battle takes on even greater significance when the hermit monk expresses his admiration for those like the archbishop who, rather than fleeing the world, elect to combat its temptations in the hope of saving it:

Ah! gardez-vous de jamais comparer le Chrétien qui n'évite les tentations qu'en les fuyant, avec celui qui leur résiste, et demeure dans le monde pour le sauver: celui-ci, rempli d'un zèle divin, risque chaque jour son salut pour celui de ses frères; le second, plein d'une craintive défiance, en ne s'occupant que du sien, ne sert à celui de personne; l'un s'expose sans cesse, combat sans relâche, triomphe toujours, croit n'avoir jamais assez fait quand il lui reste quelque chose à faire, et par la multiplicité de ses oeuvres et l'ardeur de sa foi, est un exemple vivant d'édification et de sainteté qui doit lui attirer la reconnaissance et la bénédiction de l'univers: l'autre, dans sa solitude, n'ayant aucune occasion de faillir, ne doit point se glorifier de sa sagesse; il se nourrit de l'amour de Dieu, mais il n'agit point pour Dieu; il vit en paix parce qu'il vit seul et loin des hommes auxquels il est inutile; il doit être oublié de ce monde qu'il n'a point su servir.

["Ah! Don't ever compare the Christian who only avoids temptations by fleeing them with him who resists them and remains in the world in order to save it; the latter, filled with divine zeal, risks his salvation every day for that of his brothers; the former, filled with fearful distrust, by concentrating only on his own salvation, serves no one else's; the one exposes himself to danger without ceasing, fights without repose, always triumphs, never believes he has done enough as long as there is something left to do, and by the great number of his works and the fire of his faith, is a living example of understanding and holiness that should bring him the gratitude and blessing of the universe: the other, in his solitude, having no opportunity to fall, should not vaunt his wisdom; he feeds himself on the love of God, but he does not act for God; he lives in peace because he lives alone and far from others, for whom he is useless; he should be forgotten by this world, which he did not learn how to serve.] (1:150–51)

Even as Mathilde is making her confession to the hermit, thieves attack the camp and are about to capture Mathilde when Malek appears suddenly and drives them away. He has tracked Mathilde to this desert place; he now picks her up, puts her on his horse, and carries her away. Alone with him in the desert, Mathilde is plunged into the most dangerous of situations as Malek puts tremendous pressure on her to yield to his love, just this once. She finds enough strength to resist him, however, and Malek cries out that he wants to know this God who can give one the power to conquer passion. Mathilde is overcome with joy at this possible conversion and asks him if he has become a Christian. He cannot yet say for sure, not if this religion will ask him to renounce his country and turn against his brothers. The two pray silently together, then Mathilde holds the reliquary up to him and invokes God to speak to him. At this point, Malek feels something more powerful than he has ever felt before. Mathilde then declares: "Et maintenant tu es digne d'être mon époux; je jure de n'en avoir jamais d'autre que toi, je jure à ce Dieu qui en ce moment remplit de son immensité et de sa toute-puissance, et ce désert et ton coeur!" ["And now you are worthy to be my husband; I swear never to have any other than you, I swear to that God who is at this moment filling this desert and your heart with his immensity and his omnipotence!"] (1:170). Malek knows that Mathilde is now his wife in word, but God is so powerful in the desert, all passion is eliminated and any thoughts of sensual pleasure are removed from his mind. Mathilde will remain untouched by Malek until the archbishop has joined them together.

When they arrive back in Cairo, the people of the city, happy to see Malek is not dead, nevertheless blame Mathilde for all their troubles. In fact, Saladin, led by Agnès to believe that Malek is planning to marry Mathilde and by so doing gain the support of the Christians for his regime in Egypt, has now put a price on his own brother's head. Saladin dispatches Metchoub with twelve thousand men to capture Malek; the plan is to put him in chains and, before executing him, to make him watch as Mathilde is turned over to the people of Cairo.

Malek decides to have Montmorency, one of Richard's finest soldiers, escort Mathilde back to the Christian camp. In so doing, he tells Montmorency that he is turning his wife over to him, a statement that stuns the Christian knight. Mathilde corrects Malek, saying that she is not his wife because she will only marry a Christian, but she also declares that she will never give herself to any other man. At this point, the narrator comments: "la raison peut bien nous montrer la route de la vertu, mais la religion seule donne la force d'y marcher" ["reason can show us the path of virtue, but only religion gives us the strength to walk it"] (1:183).

Agnès, now at the head of a Saracen army by order of Saladin, intercepts Montmorency's contingent on its way to Ptolemais. Montmorency dies in the ensuing battle, but Mathilde is saved and the Saracens repulsed. The joy of the Christian camp at the return of Mathilde and her escort quickly turns to sorrow at the sight of Montmorency's coffin; the great hero is buried near Ptolemais. Meanwhile, in Caesarea, the brothers Saladin and Malek are reconciled, and Saladin promises Malek that he can have Mathilde for his queen and reign as king of Jerusalem. Saladin reasons that having a Christian queen on the throne should appease the Christians. When Saladin's envoy announces this proposal to the Christian leaders, Richard is outraged and promises the hand of Mathilde to whoever kills Malek. As all swear to do so, Mathilde faints. Later, she declares to the archbishop: "je sens que, si Malek Adhel devait être rejeté de Dieu, je voudrais en être rejetée aussi" ["I feel that, if Malek Adhel were to be rejected by God, I would want to be rejected by Him also"] (1:238). Horrified, the archbishop exclaims that she should weep the rest of her life for having preferred a man to God.

A dream in which she sees Malek killed and condemned to hell, cursing her for letting him get killed when in a few days he would have converted, compels Mathilde to decide that she must tell Richard the truth. The story of the vow made in the desert appalls her brother, and he exclaims he will get the pope to break it.

When Saladin's letter of terms arrives, the Christian nobles, tempted by his offer to allow Christians freedom of worship throughout the Holy Land if Mathilde is allowed to marry Malek, vote to let a council of bishops decide the issue. Encouraged by this news, Mathilde cannot contain her joy: "elle ne retient plus sa tendresse; aimer Malek Adhel est la félicité suprême, la céleste volupté des anges; aimer Malek Adhel est la seule éternité qu'elle demanderait, il lui semble que s'il n'obtenait pas comme elle, et près d'elle, un bonheur sans fin, Dieu lui-même n'aurait pas le pouvoir de la rendre heureuse. Jamais elle n'a laissé prendre une telle licence à ses sentiments; ils sont de la passion, et ses chastes voiles sont trempés des larmes de l'amour" ["she no longer keeps her love in check; to love Malek Adhel is supreme happiness, the heavenly delight of the angels; to love Malek Adhel is the only eternity she seeks, it seems that if he did not find endless happiness like her and with her, God himself would not have the power to make her happy. Never had she given such free rein to feelings of pure passion, and tears of love wet her innocent veils"] (1:251–52).

When Malek, disguised, shows up in Mathilde's room, he asks her what she will do if the council votes to reject Saladin's offer. She repeats her vow to him, but he says that is not enough; she must vow to be his, without any other conditions. She says she will, then takes his hand, places it on the Bible and asks: "Es-tu à mon Dieu?" ["Do you belong to my God?"] (1:261). As he vacillates, a servant enters to warn them that Lusignan is on his way, and Malek is ushered out quickly, without being able to answer Mathilde's question. Later, at a dance attended by both Christians and Muslims under truce, Mathilde passes a key and a note to Malek without Lusignan seeing. Malek is stunned; could this possibly be the thing he has dreamed of for so long? Like Malek, the reader imagines that the key is to her bedchamber. In the note, however, Mathilde proposes to see him the next morning "où reposent les cendres du grand Montmorency" ["where lie the great Montmorency's ashes"] (1:276). The narrator informs us that Mathilde has only the purest intentions in arranging this meeting with Malek: "Cependant, malgré la pureté, j'ai presque dit la sainteté de ses intentions, quand le jour naît, et que le moment d'aller joindre Malek Adhel approche, sa pudeur s'étonne et s'alarme; elle hésite, elle balance: et c'est bien plus le devoir que l'amour qui lui donne le courage de partir" ["Nevertheless, despite the purity, I almost said the holiness of her intentions, when dawn arrives, and the moment to meet Malek Adhel approaches, her sense of decency is shocked and alarmed; she hesitates, she wavers: and it is duty far more than love that gives her the courage to leave"] (1:276).

When she arrives at the tomb, she is in a terrible state, wondering whether she has really done it for God or for love. Telling all her servants to wait outside while she prays inside for the conversion of the infidels, she proceeds to unlock the door and let herself in. Malek is indeed there waiting for her; as he attempts to take her in his arms, she resists, saying: "Malek Adhel, vous devez croire que ce n'est point pour écouter votre amour, ni pour nous livrer à de tendres joies, que je suis venue ici; ce serait profaner les tombeaux, insulter à la mort. Les paroles qu'on fait entendre auprès d'un cercueil doivent être saintes, sévères, et solennelles comme lui" ["Malek Adhel, you must know that I did not come here to hear of your love or have the pleasure of being together; to do so would be to defile these tombs and insult death. The words one speaks near a grave should be like it: holy, austere, and solemn"] (1:278).

This encounter of two lovers in a tomb can only make us remember similar scenes in Cottin's earlier novels, beginning with the shocking episode of Claire and Frédéric on the steps of Claire's father's tomb, followed by the scene in *Amélie* when Amélie visits her father's tomb. Both of these earlier scenes involved a heroine openly revolting before the symbolic presence of the Father and his authority. In *Mathilde*, however, passion is made to cower before the heroine's holiness; any voluptuous thoughts Malek may have had are wiped away by her look. He kneels down before her: "ô fille du ciel! tu m'ouvres un nouveau monde où je sens qu'il y a quelque chose de mieux que le plaisir;

et où la vertu a une volupté supérieure à celle de l'amour même; Mathilde, si vous n'êtes pas une femme unique, s'il y en a d'autres qui vous ressemblent en Europe, je ne m'étonne plus des hommages qu'on leur rend et de l'empire qu'elles y exercent. Comment ne pas voir une créature toute divine dans la beauté à laquelle on ne peut plaire qu'à force de gloire et de vertus?" ["O daughter of heaven! you open up a new world to me where I feel there is something better than pleasure; and where virtue has a greater attraction than love itself; Mathilde, if you are not unique, if there are others like you in Europe, I am not surprised at the honor given them there and the power they wield. How can one not see the divine beauty of a creature whom one pleases only through glorious and virtuous acts?"] (1:280). The two of them kneel at Montmorency's tomb, and Mathilde implores the spirit of Montmorency to speak to God on behalf of Malek's soul; Malek, too, prays to Montmorency, asking him to teach him how to reconcile "l'honneur, l'amitié et l'amour" ["honor, friendship, and love"] (1:281).

When the archbishop surprises Mathilde and Malek in the tomb, he asks Mathilde to come with him: "je veux que vous mesuriez vous-même la profondeur de l'abîme où les passions peuvent entraîner, et quel châtiment Dieu réserve aux coupables qui y tombent" ["I want you to see for yourself the depth of the abyss toward which the passions can lead and what punishment God reserves for the guilty who fall therein"] (1:315). He takes her to see Agnès, now completely insane, and Mathilde witnesses her rolling in the dirt, crying out the names of Malek and Mathilde. Guillaume points out that seduction caused Agnès's suffering and that he has now found Mathilde with the same man who had seduced Agnès: "Et dans quel lieu vous ai-je trouvée! continua-t-il encore, dans quel lieu l'aveuglement de l'amour a-t-il pu vous entraîner! auprès d'un tombeau! comme s'il n'y avait que son silence qui ne vous fît pas entendre de reproche. Eh quoi! ne vous disait-il rien, ce silence? pour vous la mort n'a-t-elle pas de voix? et pendant que vous la braviez, cette mort redoutable, si elle vous avait frappée; si vous étiez expirée auprès de Malek Adhel avec les mots d'amour dans la bouche et dans le coeur, où seriez-vous maintenant?" ["'And where did I find you!' he continued, 'where has the blindness of love led you! to a tomb! As if its silence alone kept you from hearing any reproach. And what! this silence, didn't it tell you anything? Does death not speak to you? And while you were defying it, this awful death, if it had struck you, if you had died near Malek Adhel with words of love on your lips and in your heart, where would you be now?'"] (1:318). At this point in the narrative, the old woman assigned to watch Agnès brings Mathilde a drink of water and asks if she will be staying with "the other."

Indeed Agnès is Mathilde's "other," the case of an extreme passion run rampant. Through her, Cottin implies that the end result of unchecked passion is madness. Apparently, the archbishop's lesson has its intended effect, for Mathilde asks Malek to take her to the convent of Carmel and the narrator comments, "Pour trouver dans son coeur la force de renoncer à la plus ardente passion, il faut bien y trouver quelque chose de plus puissant qu'elle et de supérieur à ses voluptés: la passion est beaucoup assurément, et ses voluptés des délices; mais ce sont les délices de la terre, et quiconque les sacrifie, en conçoit donc de plus ravissants encore; autrement, pourquoi les sacrifierait-il?" ["To find the strength in one's heart to give up the strongest of passions, something more powerful, something superior to its pleasures must be found: passion is certainly wonderful and its pleasures delightful; but they are delights of the world, and whoever gives them up conceives of better ones; otherwise, why give them up?"] (1:324).

Richard receives a letter from Mathilde informing him that she has retired to the monastery to escape his rule and a forced marriage. Enraged, Richard sends Guillaume and Bérengère to Carmel to tell Mathilde that if in eight days she has not taken her vows, he will force her to marry Lusignan. By subterfuge, Mathilde is finally brought back to the Christian camp to await her fate.

When the Christians attack Ascalon, a Saracen stronghold, Lusignan and Malek finally meet on the battlefield to fight to the death. They wound one another seriously and Malek drops his sword to take his dagger and kill Lusignan, but Lusignan fades so quickly in his arms that he does not strike. Lusignan's squire, who has followed them, thinking his lord is dead, thrusts his sword into Malek's neck. Malek, surprised, turns and falls. Upon his return to the Christian camp, the squire announces to Mathilde that Malek is dead; the archbishop, however, convinces Mathilde that Malek might be alive still, and the two leave the camp under cover of night to find him. When they do, he is indeed alive, but barely; the archbishop baptizes him and Malek kisses the cross: "aussitôt la lumière divine et l'abondante vie qui la suit descendent par torrents dans son âme, il aime et il croit" ["at that moment the divine light and the abundant life that follows it descended in a rush into his soul, he loves and he believes"] (1:378). Malek tells Mathilde he will wait for her; the archbishop joins their hands and calls them husband and wife. Malek dies, but Mathilde is peaceful; her wish had been that Malek become Christian. God has granted that wish, and she can ask for nothing more. Mathilde will not let go of the body and even convinces Saladin to allow her to take it with her to Carmel. The narrative describes Mathilde as "morte au monde comme l'époux qu'elle suit" ["dead to the world like the spouse she follows"] (1:385). When they arrive at Carmel, Mathilde participates in the ritual that symbolizes that she has become "dead" to the world; they cut off her hair and cover her with funeral drapery. Mathilde then has a vision of Malek in the bosom of God, which makes her supremely happy. The spirit is so strong that the Muslims who have accompanied the funeral cortege are converted, and all present become one people and of one heart. The last scene is of Mathilde watching from the convent as a boat sails for England: "elle restait seule dans l'Orient, sans famille, sans liens" ["she remained alone in the Orient, without family, without ties"] (1:398).

In *Mathilde*, the virtues of religion are praised, especially its power to control human passion, to keep emotions within bounds and, by so doing, eliminate the possibility of extreme behaviors and their attendant negative consequences. But virtue does not always have its reward, at least not in this life, for Mathilde's efforts to convert Malek, though successful, do not guarantee she will taste the felicity she longs for. In the end she is left alone and without family. Would Mathilde have been happier, in the end, if she had remained in her convent, oblivious to the cares and turmoil of the outside world? By the end of the novel, she is isolated in a foreign land, without the moral support of family and friends. She has avoided the madness of Agnès, but she may not be any happier. The message of the text is that the good and the bad are destined alike to suffer. Perhaps it is more accurate to say that according to this text, exceptional people are more likely to suffer than others; those who love in a rage, those who are stunningly beautiful, those who are as ferocious as lions, those who attempt to follow the strictest code of conduct—these norm-breakers seem especially marked out by destiny for suffering. At one point in the text, the narrator philosophizes:

> Sans doute, si la peine nous fait plus vivre que le plaisir, c'est qu'elle développe davantage et met plus en exercice tous les sentiments de notre coeur et les facultés de notre esprit. Dans la peine, la vie tout

entière est devant nous: le passé avec ses regrets, le présent avec ses larmes, l'avenir avec ses espérances; nous nous attendrissons sur nous-mêmes, nous sommes plus chers à ce qui nous entoure, et, en étant plus aimés, nous devenons meilleurs. C'est dans la peine que l'imagination s'élève aux grandes pensées de l'éternité et de la justice suprême, et qu'elle nous jette sans cesse hors de nous pour chercher un remède à nos maux. Dans le bonheur, nous sommes plus tranquilles; mais être tranquilles, être heureux, n'est pas notre destination sur la terre, et j'oserai même dire que ce n'est pas notre penchant. Ah! si la douleur attire le coeur de l'homme, s'il sent que c'est là son élément, c'est qu'elle n'a été donnée qu'à lui, c'est que seul, parmi les créatures, il a reçu le privilège de souffrir, et qu'il est fier de ce privilège, parce qu'il en aperçoit le but; car, je le demande, si Dieu n'avait pas jeté le malheur sur la terre, comment y aurait-il placé la vertu?

[Undoubtedly, if suffering, more than pleasure, makes us feel alive, it is because more than anything else it develops and stimulates all the feelings of our heart and the faculties of our mind. In suffering, all of life is before us: the past with its regrets, the present with its tears, the future with its hopes; we are moved to self-pity, we become dearer to those around us, and, in being more loved, we become better. It is in suffering that the imagination rises to great thoughts about eternity and supreme justice and it forces us unceasingly outside of ourselves to seek a remedy for our ills. In happiness, we are more at peace; but to be at peace, to be happy, is not our destiny on earth, and I will even dare say that it is not our inclination. Ah! if suffering appeals to the heart of man, if he feels that there he is in his element, it is because he alone, of all creatures, has received the privilege of suffering, and how proud he is of this privilege, because he sees the reason for it; for, I ask you, if God had not placed misfortune in the world, how would he have put virtue there?] (1:242)

The recognition that there are powers greater than oneself running the universe, powers that can allow us to suffer, like Job, in spite of our innocence and our own ignorance, is a moral typical of the Old Testament writers, and the text appears to agree with Job that suffering brings wisdom the sufferer could not have achieved in any other way. In *Claire d'Albe* and in *Amélie Mansfield*, there had been anger and revolt; in *Mathilde*, these have been supplanted by a calm resignation to submit to the Father's will.

Cottin was so encouraged by the public's reception of *Mathilde* that a week after its publication, she proclaimed to Julie, in hyperbolic language she most likely wanted to believe herself: "si j'en crois les voix qui retentissent à mes oreilles, *Mathilde* a un grand succès: on ne parle que d'elle, on ne s'occupe que d'elle, c'est le seul livre qu'on rencontre, qu'on lit partout. Les uns y trouvent bien un peu trop de *religion*, les autres un peu trop d'*épopée*, mais néanmoins les littérateurs l'estiment infiniment davantage que mes autres ouvrages, parce que les romans en général ne sont pas comptés parmi les ouvrages de littérature, et que celui-ci doit y être admis" ["If I can believe the voices resounding in my ear, *Mathilde* is a great success: people are talking of nothing else, nothing else occupies their attention, it is the only book you see, the only one being read everywhere. Some find a little too much *religion* in it, others a little too much *epic*, but nevertheless the critics admire it infinitely more than my other works, because novels in general are not considered literary works, and this one ought to be admitted into that circle"] (*MC*, 395). Obviously, with *Mathilde*, Cottin felt she had broken free of the stigma of the woman's novel and had entered the field of "true" literature—that is, the field of masculine literature, accepted and promoted by the dominant cultural paradigm. Her acceptance into that select group had been greatly aided by the collaboration of Michaud, who, as her publisher, had insisted on providing his own detailed history of the Crusades as a preface to the novel. His editorial intervention and filtering made this the most commercially successful while at the same time the least idiosyncratic of Cottin's works. *Mathilde* indeed marks Cottin's return to the mainstream.

6
Filial Devotion in *Elisabeth*

ON 28 FEBRUARY 1805, JULIE VERDIER'S HUSBAND DIED IN TONNEINS; needing to oversee the settlement of the estate, Julie left for Tonneins in early March, confiding the care of her daughters once again to their adoptive mother, Sophie. The absence stretched to six months, during which Cottin stayed hard at work revising the *Mathilde* manuscript for publication. Her letters to Julie from the time show her continued enthusiasm for the writer's craft, which had clearly become for her a therapeutic activity : "Il y a pour moi un charme dans la composition que je ne peux t'exprimer. Je m'amuse cent fois plus à méditer un sujet, à écrire quelques pages, qu'à voir Mme Hocquart jouer Zénobie, ou Mme Mallet défigurer Philaminte. Je trouve même dans ce genre de travail une séduction dont je ne me défends pas toujours sans effort. . . . Il faut bien que le charme que je trouve à composer soit véritablement très vif, car je puis dire que les jouissances de l'amour-propre étant assez faibles, ce ne sont pas elles qui l'animent" ["I cannot express how delightful writing is for me. I find a hundred times more pleasure in thinking about a topic and writing a few pages than in watching Mme. Hocquart play the role of Zénobie, or Mme. Mallet make a disaster of Philaminte. I even find a seduction in this type of work, which I do not successfully resist without quite an effort. . . . The pleasure I find in writing must be very considerable indeed, for I can say that the rewards to my vanity being so negligible, they are not the motivating force behind it"] (*MC*, 394). In another letter to Julie, she rhapsodized: "Je ne puis exprimer le plaisir que je trouve dans la composition d'un ouvrage" ["I cannot describe the pleasure I find in composing a work"] (396).

Although she extolled the joys of writing, Cottin nevertheless had to deal with the disturbing notoriety associated with the profession. After the publication of *Mathilde*, for instance, rumors began to spread that Cottin had converted to Catholicism. Writing to Azaïs about this, she complained: "Tout le mal vient de ce que je suis trop connue; j'éprouve tous les jours qu'une femme gâte bien son sort en sortant de l'obscurité: vous savez bien que, là où il y a de la peine, il y a toujours un tort; c'en est un très grand pour une femme que d'écrire; on ne saurait trop le répéter, ni moi assez le reconnaître. Mes moindres démarches sont observées, et le blâme qu'on y jette rejaillit sur ce qui m'entoure et qui m'est cher" ["All this trouble comes from the fact that I am too well known; every day I am reminded that a woman ruins her life by losing her anonymity: you know well that, where there is pain, there has always been some mistake made; it is a grave mistake for a woman to write; one cannot repeat it too often, nor can I acknowledge the fact enough. The most insignificant things I do are closely observed, and the criticism they elicit reflects on those who are near and dear to me"] (*UO*, 282). To counter all the rumors, Cottin decided she would go with Julie's daughters the next time they took communion at the Protestant church and join them in all the ceremonies. On this point, Cottin was adamant, considering it a necessity for mothers to transmit to their daughters the faith inherited from their ancestors: "L'esprit d'innovation, si dangereux parmi les hommes, est sans excuse pour les femmes; et les jeunes filles qu'on verrait élevées dans cet esprit-là seraient jugées avec une grande sévérité" ["The desire to change things, so dangerous in men, is without excuse in women; and girls seen as having been raised with that attitude would be judged harshly"] (283).

In this context, Cottin now had to come to terms with Azaïs and his philosophy, which she had so eagerly and openly embraced while in Bagnères. Azaïs himself arrived in Paris in the fall of 1806 to begin the public revelation of his philosophical system; upon his arrival, he published a synopsis of his work, *Essai sur le monde*, which the intellectual community in Paris either received with less than enthusiasm or simply ignored. Cottin, for her part, seemed anxious to distance herself from any perceived connection with his system: "Mon ami, depuis que je pratique, autant qu'il m'est possible, le devoir de mère, je sens presque que ce sera une nécessité, une loi impérieuse pour moi de ne pas adopter hautement vos idées, jusqu'au moment du moins où elles seront adoptées généralement" ["My friend, since I fulfill, as far as it is possible for me, the duties of a mother, I feel that it will be almost obligatory, even an absolute requirement for me, not to adopt your ideas openly, until the time at least when they become generally accepted"] (*UO*, 283). This decision, she maintained, was based on her belief that women should function as the guardians of tradition in society: "C'est surtout pour les femmes que c'est un devoir de première nécessité de croire à la foi de leurs pères et de ne pas la changer contre la foi d'un seul homme. Que d'abus si on lui donnait une pareille licence! Mon ami, dois-je en donner l'exemple, je vous le demande, moi malheureusement trop connue par mes ouvrages et presque mère de famille?" ["One of woman's primordial responsibilities is to adhere to the faith of her fathers and not to trade it for that of any particular man. What evils would arise from giving her such freedom! My friend, should I set the precedent for this, I ask you, I who am unfortunately too well known because of my books and almost the mother of a family?"] (283–84).

Her rejection of Azaïs's system mirrored an emotional distancing from the man himself. She was willing to acknowledge their friendship but nothing more: "Vous êtes malade, passionné et malheureux, vous êtes l'objet de ma plus tendre amitié; ne me demandez pas d'autre sentiment, mon coeur n'en peut plus éprouver d'autre" ["You are ill, passionate, and unhappy, I have a tender affection for you as a friend; don't expect any other kind of feeling from me, my heart can no longer hold any other"] (*MC*, 368). Friendship and religion, she claimed, would be from that moment on the only two interests in her life: "chaque nouveau jour ajoute une force de plus à mes sentiments de piété; mon âme se calme, s'apaise, la terre et ses biens s'effacent; mon ancre est jetée dans le ciel, je ne crains plus les tempêtes" ["each new day adds more strength to my religious devotion; my soul is growing calmer, quieter, the world and its attractions grow dim; my anchor is fixed in the heavens, I no longer fear the storms"] (368). She invited Azaïs to leave behind his self-created system and return with her to his traditional faith: "Mon ami, revenez avec moi vers ce séjour de toute lumière, de toute félicité; attachez-vous à lui, ne vous attachez qu'à lui; le coeur qui y a placé toutes ses espérances ne peut être déchiré ni trompé" ["My friend, return with me to that life full of light and happiness; embrace that and only that; the heart that has placed all its hopes there cannot be broken or deceived"] (368).

The return to the faith of her fathers that Cottin mentions here would find expression in her last published novel, *Elisabeth; ou, Les exilés de Sibérie*, a work that portrays, in the words of Madame de Genlis, "les sentimens [*sic*] les plus purs, l'amour maternel, l'amour filial" ["the purest of feelings, maternal love, filial love"] (365). It became the most popular of all of Cottin's novels, with at least forty-eight different editions in French appearing either as individual publications or in collections. In addition, *Elisabeth* was translated into English, Spanish, Portuguese, Italian, and Croatian; it has the distinction of being the most popular of Cottin's texts with the American reading public. The novel's relative brevity—67 pages in Ledentu's edition of the *Oeuvres complètes* as opposed to *Mathilde*'s 388 pages—may account in part for its publishing record. A closer look at the record, however, reveals that the key was its thematic content: because of its recognition as a "moral" tale, the story became very popular as a text for study in schools (*MC*, 415). This explains why, out of all her novels, *Elisabeth* was especially attractive to puritanical America.

Where Cottin had relied on her imagination to create her previous heroines, the story of *Elisabeth* was evidently drawn from a reportedly true story that had appeared in at least four different Parisian publications in the year 1805.[1] She apparently began work on her own version of the story in late fall 1805, after completing the *Mathilde* manuscript. We can only speculate as to why she was interested in recasting this story in her own words. In some important ways, it was an extension of the themes traced out in *Mathilde*; with *Elisabeth*, however, familial relationships replaced forbidden love as the central focus, and the story became a suitable vehicle through which Cottin publicly reaffirmed her allegiance to Father's order.

Like *Mathilde*, *Elisabeth* is composed in zero focalization. The opening description of Siberia and the circle of Ischim as the "Italy of Siberia" is skillfully done and may be Cottin's most successful descriptive passage of any of her novels. It is evidence that Cottin's abilities as a writer were improving with each new challenge; where she had once avoided long descriptive passages because of her perception that they tended only to bore the reader, she now had confidence that, when justified by the narrative's direction, a well-written description could enhance the power of the text. Certainly, in this case, where the landscape itself—Siberia—plays such a major role in the drama, Cottin felt obligated to create a persuasive word picture of the setting—and with happy results.

From Tobolsk, the capital of Siberia, to Ischim, there stretches a range of villages in which political exiles are condemned to live. In the middle of a forest, not far from the village of Saïmka, lives a family of three: a father, a mother, and a beautiful young daughter. They communicate with no one except a poor peasant woman who works as their servant. No one knows their homeland, their lineage, or the cause of their punishment. Only the governor of Tobolsk knows their secret, and he has informed his lieutenant in Saïmka that the family is to have no communication with the outside world, particularly with the Russian court. Because of the special attention paid him by the officials, the people of Saïmka assume that Pierre Springer—the name given to the exile—descends from an illustrious and wealthy family and is therefore either guilty of a great crime or the victim of a great injustice. Curiosity about his case, however, wanes as time passes, and the family is eventually forgotten by the locals. Springer spends his days hunting and trapping in the forest; the sale of ermine furs allows him to procure decent furniture brought from Tobolsk as well as books for his daughter's education. The long Siberian evenings are spent instructing Elisabeth, the father specializing in tales of glory and heroism, the mother Phédora in moral and religious training. The result, the text tells us, is "un caractère courageux, sensible, qui, réunissant l'extraordinaire énergie de Springer à l'angélique douceur de Phédora, fut tout à la fois noble et fier comme tout ce qui vient de l'honneur, et tendre et dévoué comme tout ce qui vient de l'amour" ["a courageous and sensitive character which, uniting the extraordinary energy of Springer with Phédora's angelic sweetness, was both noble and proud, like all things nourished by honor, and tender and devoted, like everything that grows out of love"] (1:476). In the spring, the family works the garden; Springer has built a greenhouse in which he raises the flowers of his homeland. When they bloom, he adorns his daughter's hair with them and says to her: "Elisabeth, pare-toi des fleurs de ta patrie, elles te ressemblent; comme toi elles s'embellissent dans l'exil. Ah! puisses-tu n'y pas mourir comme elles!" ["Elisabeth, adorn yourself with the flowers of your fatherland, they resemble you; like you, they grow more beautiful in exile. Ah! may you not die there as they will do!"] (1:476).

Outside of these rare moments of expressed emotion, Springer remains quiet and somber, sitting for hours without a word, pensive, his eyes directed toward a particular point on the horizon and his chest heaving in great sighs. He reproaches his wife for her decision to share his exile, but she claims she could never know happiness apart from him. In fact, she points out, as exiles, they now have more time to spend together than ever in their former life.

Elisabeth has grown up in the woods and has no recollection of any other home; she cannot imagine a life more wonderful than her own: "Ainsi, loin du monde et des hommes, croissait en beauté cette jeune vierge pour les yeux seuls de ses parents, pour l'unique charme de leur coeur: semblable à la fleur du désert, qui ne s'épanouit qu'en présence du soleil, et ne se pare pas moins de vives couleurs, quoiqu'elle ne puisse être vue que par l'astre à qui elle doit la vie" ["Thus, far from the world and humanity, this young virgin grew in beauty for the admiration of her parents only, a joy to their hearts alone: like the desert flower that blossoms only in the presence of the sun and yet adorns itself in brilliant colors, though the star that gave it life is the only thing that may gaze upon it"] (1:478). Elisabeth loves her parents deeply: "ils étaient tout pour elle: les protecteurs de sa faiblesse, les compagnons de ses jeux, et son unique société" ["they were everything to her: her protectors, her playmates, and her only social circle"] (1:478). Everything she knows, she knows thanks to them. When she grows old enough to become aware of her parents' perpetual sadness, she inquires of them the cause of their condition. Upon learning that they live in exile, Elisabeth resolves to make the one goal of her life the restoration of her parents to their homeland.

This, then, becomes the narrative's central driving plot element: to succeed, Elisabeth must go to St. Petersburg to ask the emperor in person to pardon her father. It will be no small task, as it is a journey of over two thousand miles, most of which must be made on foot. This heroic effort symbolizes the depth of her devotion to the father. Her will, courage, and confidence in God reassure her she can do it, but she cannot even begin without the help of a guide. Elisabeth remembers a young man, Smoloff, the son of the governor of Tobolsk who, while on a bear hunt, had once saved her father's life; thinking that he may be the link she needs, she resolves to find a way to contact him.

Providence provides her with the desired opportunity. One cold winter day, Springer leaves to hunt. The two women, fearing for his life after the episode with the bear, decide to go after him. After trudging through the snow for hours, Phédora's strength gives out, and her stronger daughter, "élevée dans ces climats et accoutumée à braver les froids les plus rigoureux" ["raised in this climate and accustomed to braving the most bitter cold"], tells her to stay and rest (1:481). Elisabeth pushes on until she arrives at the steppes, where she hears a gunshot and thinks it must be her father but discovers instead a handsome young hunter. He is struck by the courage, tenderness, and pain reflected in her eyes: "il croyait rêver, il n'avait rien vu, jamais rien imaginé de pareil à Elisabeth" ["he thought he was dreaming, he had never seen or imagined anything like Elisabeth"] (1:482). When he discovers she is the daughter of the man he once saved, he is overwhelmed. He assures her that her father is on his way home; Elisabeth hurries to find her mother, and the two women make their way back to their hut. Upon arriving home, Elisabeth is surprised to find that the young man has followed them. The father introduces him to the two women as his savior, and they fall at his feet in gratitude. Because nightfall is near, Smoloff must stay with them, though it is forbidden by his own father's orders. The narrative allows us to see Elisabeth through Smoloff's eyes: "La simplicité de son costume semblait rehausser encore la dignité de son maintien, et tous ses mouvements étaient accompagnés d'une grâce que Smoloff admirait avec une singulière émotion, et dont il ne pouvait détacher ni ses regards, ni son coeur" ["Her simplicity of dress seemed to emphasize once again the dignity of her demeanor, and everything she did was characterized by a grace that Smoloff admired with uncommon emotion and from which he found it impossible to avert his eyes or his heart"] (1:483). Elisabeth looks at him in turn, but her gaze is fundamentally different: "Elisabeth ne le regardait pas avec moins de plaisir; mais dans ce plaisir tout était pur; il ne venait que de la reconnaissance qu'elle lui devait, et des espérances qu'elle fondait sur lui" ["Elisabeth found no less pleasure in looking at him, but in this pleasure all was pure; it came only from the gratitude she felt and the hope she placed in him"] (1:483). The narrative makes it clear that Elisabeth is motivated purely by filial affection: "Dieu lui-même, qui sonde jusqu'aux derniers replis du coeur, n'aurait pas trouvé dans celui d'Elisabeth un seul sentiment qui ne se rapportât à ses parents, et qui ne fût entièrement pour eux" ["God himself, who sees into the deepest recesses of the heart, would not have found a single feeling in Elisabeth's heart unrelated to her parents and their welfare"] (1:483).

Springer expresses his sorrow for the situation he has placed his daughter in: "Jamais tu ne jouiras de ce plaisir que je te dois, jamais la voix d'un enfant adoré ne te fera entendre de si douces paroles: tu vivras seule ici, sans époux, sans famille, comme un faible oiseau égaré dans le désert. Innocente victime, tu ne connais point les biens que tu perds; mais moi, qui ne peux plus te les donner, j'ai tout perdu" ["You will never enjoy the happiness I should have given you, you will never hear a beloved child's voice saying such sweet words: you will live here alone, without a husband, without a family, like a fragile bird lost in the wilderness. An innocent victim, you don't know the wonderful things you are being deprived of; but I, who can no longer give them to you, I have lost everything"] (1:484). Smoloff says that he has seen many exiles forced to live without friends or family; Springer acknowledges then, as he takes his daughter's hand, that indeed he has not lost everything.

When Smoloff leaves the following morning, Elisabeth is disappointed that she has not had the chance to talk to him about her plans. She asks him to return, and he replies that he will try to get an exception from his father to visit them. Phédora asks him to see if his father will grant her the permission to attend church services with Elisabeth each Sunday. The narrator describes the thoughts of Smoloff as he leaves: "il se persuada que la rencontre de la veille n'était pas un coup du hasard, qu'une mutuelle sympathie avait agi sur Elisabeth comme sur lui, et il était impatient de lire dans ce coeur innocent la confirmation de tout ce qu'il osait espérer" ["he was convinced that the encounter of the preceding day had not been a mere accident, that he and Elisabeth had felt a mutual attraction, and he was anxious to read in that innocent heart the confirmation of all he dared hope for"] (1:485). But the narrator interjects at this point: "Ah! qu'il était loin de deviner ce qu'il devait y lire un jour!" ["Oh! how far he was from guessing correctly what he would one day find there!"] (1:485). Smoloff has misread and misinterpreted the behavior of Elisabeth; the "mutual attraction" he believes is motivating her is in actuality love for her father.

Elisabeth, now seventeen years old, asks her father to tell her what she needs to know in order to help him. He perceives that she is planning to do something, and he is already immensely relieved and grateful. But he asks her to give him some time before he makes his revelation. He delays beyond what she had expected; in the meantime, she strengthens herself for her anticipated ordeal by walking every day on the flats in every sort of weather imaginable. One day, a ferocious storm forces her to take refuge in a small wooden chapel, where she falls asleep lying in front of the altar. In the meantime, Smoloff returns to their home with the good news that Phédora and Elisabeth will be allowed to attend church on Sundays. The bad news, however, is that this will be the last time he is permitted to visit them. When the storm strikes, Smoloff and Springer leave the safety of the hut to find Elisabeth. When they discover her in the chapel, she informs them that she is ready to leave: "elle est fière de ses forces; elle éprouve une sorte d'orgueil à les montrer à son père; elle espère le convaincre qu'elle n'en manquera point pour aller chercher sa grâce, fallût-il aller la chercher à l'autre extrémité du monde" ["she is proud of her strength; she feels a sort of pride in demonstrating it for her father; she hopes to convince him that she does not lack the strength to seek his pardon, even if she has to go to the other end of the world to find it"] (1:492).

The narrative continues to reinforce the juxtaposition of filial and romantic love as it ironically describes the series of misinterpretations Smoloff gives to Elisabeth's actions. When Elisabeth learns that this will be Smoloff's last visit, for instance, she appears troubled. He once again interprets this as interest in him whereas, as the narrator points out, Elisabeth's focus is obstinately fixed on her father; she is thinking only of the difficulty now of discussing her projected journey with Smoloff. In a succeeding episode, Elisabeth closes her eyes while listening to the choir at church and, inspired by the angelic voices, feels that God must be sending a guardian angel to guide her on her way. When she opens her eyes, her gaze falls on Smoloff, who is looking at her intently; this she interprets as a sign that he will play the role of that angel. He, on the other hand, once again misreads her thankful look and is encouraged in his belief that she is interested in him. He offers to drive Elisabeth and her mother in his sleigh to the edge of the forest and, as Elisabeth descends from the sleigh, he arranges to meet her the following day in the little chapel. The innocent girl has no idea whatsoever how Smoloff has interpreted her consent to meet him there.

When Smoloff arrives at the chapel, he is surprised to find that Elisabeth has preceded him, and the narrator comments: "On va vite sans doute quand c'est la passion qui entraîne; mais Elisabeth venait de prouver en ce jour que la vertu qui court à son devoir peut aller plus vite encore" ["Love certainly quickens one's pace; but that day Elisabeth proved that goodness running to fulfill its duty goes even faster"] (1:494). When she sees him, she tells him how impatiently she has been awaiting his arrival; he again misinterprets this and is about to tell her that he too is in love when she reveals her project. Smoloff is dumbfounded but, falling to his knees, he promises to obey her. She informs him of her ferocious commitment to save her father; although disappointed about his misunderstanding of her intentions, he nevertheless greatly admires her courage and determination. She begs his help in finding a route to follow and shelter along the way and also asks that he persuade the governor not to punish her father for her attempt. Smoloff is astonished to learn that Elisabeth knows nothing of her father's former status, his alleged crime against the emperor, and the emperor's hatred of him. She is certain of only one thing: her father's innocence. Smoloff exclaims: "Ô fille étonnante! . . . pas un mouvement d'orgueil, de vanité dans ton dévouement! tu ne sais point ce que tu vas reconquérir: tu n'as pensé qu'à tes parents; mais qu'est-ce que la grandeur de ta naissance devant celle de ton âme?" ["O amazing girl that you are! . . . not an ounce of pride or vanity in your devotion! You don't know what you will regain for yourself by this: you have thought only of your parents; but what is the grandeur of your ancestry in comparison to that of your soul?"] (1:496). He tells her that he needs time to think the proposal over but that in the meantime she needs to know that he loves her and would prefer living in obscurity with her to all the honors the world could bestow.

Elisabeth has never thought of any love other than filial love; she can hardly conceive of it, since her heart is filled only with the idea of her parents' misfortunes. The narrator declares: "pour en contenir deux [passions], le coeur humain, tout vaste qu'il est, ne l'est point encore assez" ["to possess two passions, the human heart, as vast as it is, is yet not vast enough"] (1:497). The message is clear: as long as Father needs her help, there will be no room in Elisabeth's life for any other kind of attachment.

When Smoloff fails to show up at church the following Sunday as promised, Elisabeth is bitterly disappointed. The people at church, however, inform her that Smoloff had left for Tobolsk two days earlier. Elisabeth goes to church each Sunday over the next two months, each time hoping in vain to find Smoloff there. When April arrives and the weather turns springlike, she decides that in the absence of Smoloff, she will have to count on God and her own resources to carry out her plan.

She informs her father that she is leaving: "permets-moi; je le sens, c'est Dieu lui-même qui m'appelle" ["let me go; I feel it is God himself who is calling me"] (1:500). At that very moment, a servant appears, announcing the arrival of M. Smoloff. Elisabeth, believing this to be a sign that God is removing the obstacles to her plans and opening the way, is deeply disappointed to find that it is the elder Smoloff, governor of Tobolsk, who has come. The governor informs the family that two months earlier his son had received orders from the emperor to depart immediately for the army. He had left a letter with his father asking that it be delivered to the Springer family, but the governor had not found the opportunity to do so until then. Blushing, Elisabeth takes the letter to read in secret. In it, Smoloff promises to take her to St. Petersburg and introduce her to the emperor. He promises to protect her during the trip: "ne craignez point mon amour, je n'en parlerai plus, je ne serai que votre ami, que votre frère; et, si je vous sers avec toute la vivacité de la passion, je jure de ne vous parler jamais qu'un langage pur comme l'innocence, comme les anges, comme vous" ["do not fear my love, I will speak of it no more, I will only be your friend, your brother; and, if I serve you with all the intensity of passion, I swear to speak to you only in the pure language of innocence, as the angels do, as you yourself speak"] (1:503). Smoloff's dangerous romantic passion is thus sublimated into a brotherly and protective affection, putting Elisabeth at ease. But Smoloff's father suggests an even safer alternative: he will send a Christian missionary to act as guide for Elisabeth's journey as a substitute for his son. The danger of Smoloff's passion is thus further distanced from the object of its desire and there will be another "father," this time a priest, to take his place.

Elisabeth is finally introduced to her father's own hidden narrative on the following day. A potential heir to the throne of Poland, he had defended his country against Russian invasion until the very last moment. Fearing that he posed a threat, the Russian emperor had ordered him seized and imprisoned in St. Petersburg. Phédora had joined him there, where they lived in the dungeons for a year before he was exiled to Siberia for life. His wife had followed him there as well: "Si j'eusse été envoyé dans les ténèbres glacées de l'affreux Beresoff, dans les solitudes perdues du lac Baïkal ou du Kamchatka, je n'y aurais pas été seul encore; il n'est point de désert, il n'est point d'antre si sauvage où ma Phédora ne m'eût suivi" ["If I had been sent to the frozen shadows of the terrible Beresoff, into the far-flung solitude of Lake Baïkal or Kamchatka, I would have not been there alone; there is no wilderness or cavern so forbidding that it could keep my Phédora from following me"] (1:508). The challenge for Elisabeth to match or better the mother's devotion becomes obvious at this point.

When the promised missionary guide arrives, Elisabeth at last embarks on her journey; her pilgrimage will turn out to be as arduous as any conceived in the name of religious faith, but it is concern for the Father's redemption, not for her own salvation, that drives her on. During the month it takes them to cross the forests of Siberia, they find shelter with the poor, in houses reeking of smoke, brandy, and tobacco with adults, children, and animals sharing the same sleeping space. When they arrive in Perme, the largest town Elisabeth has ever seen, she is saddened by the city's narrow dirty streets and fetid air. Despite all this, Elisabeth finds the trip easier than she had imagined. By the first of September, they have reached the banks of the Kama, about 130 miles from Kasan, the halfway point in their journey. The narrator then gives a foreshadowing of the difficult trials to come: "Ah! si le ciel eût permis qu'Elisabeth l'eût fini ainsi qu'elle l'avait commencé, elle aurait cru avoir faiblement payé le bonheur d'être utile à ses parents; mais tout allait changer, et avec la mauvaise saison s'approchait le moment qui devait exercer son courage, mettre au jour sa vertu, et sur la tête du juste la couronne immortelle de vie" ["Ah! if heaven had allowed Elisabeth to finish the journey as she had begun it, she would have thought she had sacrificed very little for the happiness of helping her parents; but everything was going to change and, with the arrival of winter, the time was coming that would test her courage, reveal her virtue, and place the eternal crown of life on a worthy head"] (1:516–17).

The old missionary, growing weaker each day, finally reaches the end of his strength at Sarapoul. Elisabeth tries to concoct medicines for him, but they both know that he is near death. As her spiritual father, he announces to her prophetically:

"La crainte de Dieu et l'amour de vos parents, voilà ce qui est audessus de tout, et voilà ce que vous avez. A quelque extrémité que vous soyez réduite, vous n'abandonnerez jamais ces biens pour quelque bien qu'on puisse vous offrir, et vous vous souviendrez toujours qu'une seule faute porterait la mort au sein de ceux qui vous ont donné la vie.... Au moment de la mort, je puis vous le dire, ma fille, votre vertu est grande; le monde en voit peu de semblables, il en sera touché; elle aura sa récompense sur la terre avant de l'avoir dans le ciel."

["The fear of God and the love of your parents, these are superior to all else, and these are what you have. Whatever extremity you are reduced to, you will never abandon these good things for anything anyone could offer you, and you will always remember that a single mistake would bring death to those who gave you life.... At the brink of death, I can tell you, my daughter, your virtue is great, the kind the world sees rarely, it will be touched by yours; your virtue will have its reward on earth before it receives it in heaven."] (1:518–19)

With these words, the missionary gives her his little ebony cross and dies.

Elisabeth now must face her challenge entirely alone, a condition made even more difficult by her sex. She is well aware of the risks run by a woman traveling alone in the wilderness, but whenever fear seizes her heart, she repeats the words "Mon père, ma mère," and this calms her. Traveling very slowly, she has only made it to Kasan by the first days of October. At the River Volga, already swollen with ice floes, the boatmen refuse to take her across until the river has frozen solid, which they say will take at least two weeks. After she explains her plight to them, one consents to attempt the crossing; halfway across, he can go no further by boat and so he carries Elisabeth the rest of the way on his shoulders. Once on the other side, instead of taking her money, he gives her some of his own. Elisabeth decides to keep it to give to her father upon her return as proof that "partout une protection paternelle a veillé sur moi" ["everywhere I went a paternal protection watched over me"] (1:523). She gives her last ruble to a man headed to exile in Siberia who cannot pay the postage to notify his daughter of his fate. Elisabeth's shoes are now in shambles, her clothing tattered, and the snow is piling ever deeper.

Arriving at the edge of the forests situated between Volodimr and Pokrof, known to be infested by thieves, she decides that since she has no money anyway, she should have no fear of being robbed—and so she plunges ahead. Here Elisabeth meets the greatest test of her courage. While crossing the swamps, which have frozen solid, she falls into a partially thawed section. Covered with mud and drained of energy, she sits down to ponder her situation. Behind her is the frozen marsh—ahead of her, the endless forest. The sun is setting, and she has no shelter for the night. Suddenly, she hears men's voices and rejoices, thinking she is saved, then realizes upon seeing them that they are most likely thieves. When they spy Elisabeth, they stop to interrogate her. They are so astounded by her story that they decide to leave her unharmed. At their departure, Elisabeth runs even deeper into the forest and almost immediately finds a crossroads with a road sign indicating the direction to the next town. Her story of devotion to Father not only protects her from evil men, she is now rewarded in a miraculous way by a providential hand indicating the path to follow. There is no longer any question that her pilgrimage is a sacred one, sanctioned by heaven itself.

Following the road to Pokrof, she discovers a convent and asks asylum. The nuns admire her courage and virtue; they can offer her no money, but they give her articles of their own clothing to replace her rags. At last, Elisabeth is on the road to Moscow.

Stopping in a village along the way, she is surprised by the affluence of the travelers she sees. The sound of cannons firing from the direction of Moscow announces the arrival of the emperor in town. She is shocked to learn that he is not in St. Petersburg after all but in Moscow for the ceremony of his crowning. This appears to her as a sign from heaven once again, since national celebrations are a time when monarchs set aside justice and allow mercy to sway them. Thus, Elisabeth enters Moscow with great hopes that, after ten months of privation, her suffering will soon be at an end.

With all the visitors in town, no inn is ready to offer charity, and Elisabeth can find no place to stay. She sits down next to the great fire burning in Kremlin Square and begins to weep in silence. Pride keeps her from begging alms from passerbys, but she knows that if she does not find a place soon, she will die of exposure. The first passerby scolds her for not working and gives her nothing; others either ignore her or give her a pittance too little to pay for a room. As the fire dies down, the soldiers guarding the palace come to interrogate her. They do not believe her story and begin mocking her. She pleads with the onlookers to help her, and once again Providence steps in. One man in the crowd takes pity on her and tells the soldiers he owns an inn and will provide the poor girl a place to stay. He takes her to his home, where he relates to his wife the circumstances of their meeting. At their prompting, Elisabeth tells them her story. They weep together, and the husband and wife promise to do all they can to help her. Since she has no one to intercede officially for her, they suggest she go the next day to the emperor's coronation to throw herself at his feet and plead for her father's pardon. That night, Elisabeth can hardly sleep, thinking she is so close to realizing her dream.

The next day, wearing a dress borrowed from her benefactress, Elisabeth heads toward the Church of the Assumption, where the emperor Alexander is to be crowned. The splendor of the ceremony is dazzling. "Maître du plus vaste empire de l'univers," the priest proclaims to the emperor, "vous qui allez jurer de présider aux destinées d'un état qui contient la cinquième partie du globe, n'oubliez jamais que vous allez répondre devant Dieu du sort de tant de milliers d'hommes, et qu'une injustice faite au moindre d'entre eux, et que vous auriez pu prévenir, vous sera comptée au dernier jour" ["Master of the greatest empire in the universe, you who will swear to preside over the destinies of a state covering a fifth part of the globe, never forget that you will answer to

God for the fate of thousands of men, and that an injustice done to the least among them, which you could have prevented, will be counted against you at the last day"] (1:534). As the emperor begins to take the oath to devote his time and his life to the happiness of his people, Elisabeth, with supernatural strength, breaks through the crowd and the lines of soldiers, crying "Grâce, grâce!" Guards seize her and remove her from the church, but the emperor orders one of his officers to find out what this woman wants. That officer turns out to be none other than the young Smoloff himself, and he is astonished to see Elisabeth; she tells him she has come on foot all the way from Tobolsk. He escorts her back into the church and presents her to the emperor, explaining that she has come a great distance to plead for her father's pardon. The crowd expresses admiration for the heroic feat, and the emperor is convinced that the father of such a daughter cannot be guilty. He declares to Elisabeth that her father is pardoned, upon which she faints. When she revives, the first person she sees is Smoloff. She whispers to him that now they will see her parents happy. Her use of "we" encourages him greatly.

A few days later, Smoloff arrives with an official document, the emperor's order to Smoloff's father to free Springer, now once again called by his true name, Stanislas Potowsky. In addition, Potowsky's title and riches are to be restored. Elisabeth expresses her wish to accompany Smoloff and the courier tasked to deliver the document. She tells Smoloff that she wants him to announce the good news to her father but he insists: "Non, Elisabeth, ce bonheur sera notre partage; moi j'aspire à un plus haut prix" ["No, Elisabeth, we will share this happiness; myself, I hope for a greater prize"] (1:537). This, he says, he will tell her only once he is kneeling before her father.

On their way home, Elisabeth visits the boatman who had taken her across the Volga; she finds him bedridden and his children famished. She shows him the coin he had given her, which she has kept sacred; she then gives him a hundred rubles in gratitude. She is so anxious to get home that they travel night and day, but not without stopping to visit the grave of the missionary in Sarapoul: "il lui semblait que du haut du ciel le pauvre religieux se réjouissait de la voir heureuse, et que, dans ce coeur plein de charité, la vue du bonheur d'autrui pouvait même ajouter au parfait bonheur qu'il goûtait dans le sein de Dieu" ["it seemed to her that from heaven above the poor priest was rejoicing in seeing her happy, and that, in this heart full of charity, the sight of the happiness of others could even add to the perfect happiness he enjoyed in the bosom of God"] (1:537).

Wanting to surprise her parents, Elisabeth has not allowed anyone to notify them of her return. With only Smoloff accompanying her, she sees the little hut but hesitates, and the narrator exclaims: "Ah! misère de l'homme, te voilà bien tout entière! Nous voulons du bonheur, nous en voulons avec excès, et l'excès du bonheur nous tue; nous ne pouvons le supporter" ["Ah! wretchedness of man, there you are! We want happiness, we want it badly, and yet too much happiness kills us; we cannot bear it"] (1:538). She runs up to the house, hears voices, and calls for her parents; the door opens, she sees her father, he cries out, her mother comes, and they all embrace. Smoloff then announces: "la voilà qui vous apporte votre grâce; elle a triomphé de tout, elle a tout obtenu" ["Here is the one who brings you your pardon; she has triumphed over everything, she has regained everything"] (1:538). This news, the narrator claims, adds nothing to the parents' happiness: "absorbés dans la vue de leur fille, ils savent seulement qu'elle est revenue, qu'elle est devant leurs yeux, qu'ils l'ont retrouvée, qu'ils la tiennent, qu'ils ne la quitteront plus; ils ont oublié qu'il existe d'autres biens dans le monde.... [I]ls pleurent, ils gémissent, et leurs forces, comme leur raison, se perdent dans l'excès de leur joie" ["preoccupied by the sight of their daughter, they know only that she has returned, that she is before their eyes, that she has been restored to them, that they embrace her, that they will never again leave her; they have forgotten anything else exists in the world.... [T]hey weep, they wail, and their strength, like their reason, is swallowed up in their extreme joy"] (1:538).

Thus Elisabeth, the strong, irrepressible daughter, triumphs over all obstacles to win the release of her father. She has proven herself to the world. Obsessively devoted to his cause, she demonstrates the lengths to which a child may go in the name of filial affection. To be sure, Smoloff's love for Elisabeth will be rewarded, as she accepts his proposal of marriage—with her father's approval, of course—but love between man and woman is relegated to second tier in the face of Elisabeth's sacrifice for the father. We are obviously now a long way from *Claire d'Albe*. Where Claire had committed crimes on the steps of Father's tomb in open revolt, Elisabeth now adorns his monument with triumphal bouquets, honoring his centrality and authority in her life. It is clear that revolt has been eliminated in favor of a struggle against the forces threatening Father's happiness. Like a guardian angel for her father, Elisabeth is declared pure and perfect, the combination of love and innocence found in her, we are told, guaranteeing eternal happiness.[2]

In this story, Cottin has created no intriguing doubles to contrast with the heroine, no equivalent of *Mathilde*'s Agnès to represent a possible other side to the central character. All frailties, all possible weaknesses, have been erased from Elisabeth: despite all odds, this heroine never once wavers in her single-minded devotion to duty. Her world is a world of blacks and whites, of absolutes. As a consequence of this portrayal of humans as unidimensional personalities, the narrative moves from realism into the realm of myth, the magic story or fairy tale. Indeed Elisabeth's journey has many of the mythic properties associated with the Russian magic tale.[3] Its attraction as a pedagogic tool, a "moral tale," stems in large part from this simplistic narrative world in which evil is overcome and good rewarded. Our last image of Elisabeth is of her restored to her parents, with the happy prospects of marriage to a man she has chosen and whom her parents find worthy of her. Never before had Cottin published such a story, and it is interesting to note that, even while subscribing to the moral universe she had created around Elisabeth and believing in its ultimate victory, she could not help reminding the reader at the very end of her tale that "happy endings" are merely fictions:

> Je n'irai pas plus loin. Quand les images riantes, les scènes heureuses se prolongent trop, elles fatiguent, parce qu'elles sont sans vraisemblance: on n'y croit point, on sait trop qu'un bonheur constant n'est pas un bien de la terre. La langue, si variée, si abondante pour les expressions de la douleur, est pauvre et stérile pour celles de la joie; un seul jour de félicité les épuise. . . . Ce que j'ai connu de la vie, de ses inconstances, de ses espérances trompées, de ses fugitives et chimériques félicités, me ferait craindre, si j'ajoutais une seule page à cette histoire, d'être obligée d'y placer un malheur.

> [I will go no further. When happy images and happy scenes are prolonged too much, they fatigue us, because they lack realism: we do not believe them, we know that enduring happiness is not a property of this earth. Our language, so rich, so abundant in its ability to express sorrow, is impoverished and barren when it comes to expressing joy; a single happy day exhausts the entire reserve of such expressions. . . . What I know of life, its fickleness, its dashed hopes, its fleeting and imaginary happiness, would force me to speak of unhappiness, if I were to add a single page to this story.] (1:540)

And so the text ends not on *bonheur* but rather on *malheur*, Cottin's sobering reminder of the ephemeral nature of human happiness. In *Elisabeth*, she has created a mythic image of filial devotion, taking on the role of defender of Father's faith with all seriousness. But she is also aware that virtue often goes unrewarded and that the innocent suffer in this life. This was the real world she knew, a world that would soon impose itself on her own life again in a dramatic and tragic way, proving, as she had claimed, that "enduring happiness is not a property of this earth"(1:540).

Conclusion

Shortly after the publication of *Elisabeth*, Cottin embarked on a trip to Italy as traveling companion to her friend Mélanie Lemarcis who, most likely suffering from a type of nervous disorder, had been advised by her doctors to travel to improve her health. The two left Paris on 27 August 1806 and, passing through Geneva, Vevey, Brig, and Milan, arrived in Venice on 4 October; after only a week in Venice, they returned to Milan, where indications are that they intended to begin the return trip to France. They apparently decided to go to Rome instead, and after wandering through Bologna, Florence, Pisa, and Sienna, among others, they finally arrived in Rome on 1 November. There they stayed for nearly a month. Cottin's letters to Julie back in Paris attested to the beneficial effects of this trip on her friend but also contained indications of her strong desire to return home. She missed Julie and the children terribly; they were her "treasure," for, paraphrasing the Bible, she claimed "le vrai trésor est là où on a mis son coeur" ["the true treasure is there where your heart is"] (*MC*, 398). The return trip was begun in the first part of December; this time, the two women's itinerary took them through Modena, Turino, Lyon, and Nevers. Cottin was more than anxious to be back at Champlan: "Adieu Rome! Adieu l'Italie! Je vous quitte en vous admirant, mais je retourne à ce que j'aime, et mon coeur nage dans la joie" ["Adieu, Rome! Adieu, Italy! I leave, full of admiration for you, but I am returning to the things I love, and my heart is overflowing with joy"] (399). She was at last restored to her beloved Julie and the children in the first week of January 1807.

After her return from the trip to Italy, Cottin felt the first symptoms of the illness that would take her life. As she began to face what would prove to be her final ordeal, she declared: "Je porte en moi-même un calme ravissant, une sérénité angélique. Je suis heureuse, je suis sûre de l'être toujours, car mon bonheur n'est pas dans les événements, il est en moi. J'ai appris non seulement à me résigner, mais à aimer les peines que Dieu m'envoie.

Elles ne sont que l'expiation de mes torts et je bénis sa justice et sa bonté. Je ne m'enfoncerai jamais dans le chaos des sciences, ma piété n'a pas besoin de savoir, elle est toute d'amour" ["I carry a wonderful peace, an angelic serenity in my heart. I am happy, I am sure of always being so, for my happiness is not based on events, it is inside me. I have learned not only to resign myself to but to love the sufferings that God sends me. They are merely the atonement for my sins, and I praise his justice and goodness. I will never plunge into the chaos of the sciences, my religious devotion has no need to know, it is all love"] (*UO*, 320). In spite of her illness, she continued work on two new manuscripts: one a treatise on education and the other a religious tract entitled "Religion Proven through Sentiment," neither of which was completed before her death (318). These new projects—both nonfiction with apparent didactic objectives—appear at first to be a departure from the norm. However, when we consider the text immediately preceding these, *Elisabeth,* and the ideological ends it was made to serve, then these others seem but logical extensions of the same impulse. They are evidence of Cottin's increasingly firm resolve to use her talents to write what she believed to be inspirational and morally useful works. Perhaps this too played a part in her perceived need to "atone" for past transgressions, to make retribution for earlier texts, which had been viewed as morally subversive. Whatever the reasons, it is obvious she had reoriented her focus as a writer in the last year of her life.

Sainte-Beuve claimed that "Madame Cottin s'est tuée à Palaiseau d'un coup de pistolet dans un jardin,—comme un homme" ["Madame Cottin killed herself with a pistol shot in a garden at Palaiseau—like a man would do").[1] Sainte-Beuve had a penchant for stating hearsay as fact; perhaps, distanced historically as he was from the actual event, he mixed up Cottin's story with that of Jacques Lafargue, the frustrated young man who had committed suicide at Champlan many years earlier. Or perhaps, as was often the case, he was guilty of trying to spice up what he undoubtedly viewed as an uneventful, mundane life. In any case, Sainte-Beuve's version of Cottin's death was taken as truth for many years. The letters of Julie Verdier and her daughter, however, disprove his story.[2] Instead of a sudden, violent death, they describe a death occurring after many days of protracted agony. A recent biographer claims that Cottin died of tuberculosis—which would fit with the slow death—but, once again, like Sainte-Beuve, without any documentary evidence.[3] Assuming that this kind of malady, even under a different name, was common enough in

Cottin's day to be recognizable to the lay person, it is therefore striking that no mention of the symptoms of consumption—coughing or bloody mucus—is made in the Verdier family letters describing Cottin's last days. In fact, the letters are absolutely silent about the actual cause of death, which gives more credence to Leslie Sykes's claim that Sophie Cottin died of breast cancer.[4] Sykes bases his claim on family documents he personally consulted while researching Cottin's life, which indicated that Cottin had been operated on for breast cancer and had died from the disease. This could explain the family letters' silence about the cause of death, since it was most likely considered improper to discuss the symptoms of such an illness in a public forum. We need only remind ourselves of Cottin's embarrassment when she was forced to talk of menstruation in a letter to a man—and even then she never allowed herself to use the actual terminology.

As Edward Shorter has pointed out, a woman living in the early nineteenth century who discovered a lump in her breast had few options. She could choose to ignore it, in which case the tumor would grow and spread itself throughout the body, eventually shutting down the vital organs. The breast itself would ultimately become ulcerated. "A cancer itself has no smell, nor particular effluvium," explains Shorter, "but as it advances, the necrotic tissue around it becomes infected and produces an odorous discharge. This (in addition to pain) was one of the distinctive problems of breast cancer."[5] If a woman elected to have surgery, she had to choose between a localized, restricted procedure in which only the lump would be removed and a much more radical intervention in which the entire breast would be removed. In either case, she did not enjoy the benefits of antiseptics or anesthesia, neither of which would be developed until much later in the century. Mammectomies were performed simply by seizing the breast with large pincers and cutting it off.[6] If the woman did not die while being operated on, it was only a matter of time before either infection or the spread of the cancer took her life, since operations were rarely effective.

After three months of suffering, Sophie Cottin died on 15 August 1807 at the age of thirty-seven. In a letter to her mother, one of Julie's daughters—most likely Delphine, the eldest—described her feelings about the loss she felt at Cottin's passing: "Je pense, maman, que nous avons perdu en notre seconde mère, maman Sophie, une personne qui nous chérissait tendrement; et une chère bienfaitrice qui a répandu milles douceurs sur notre vie, depuis que nous existons, à qui nous devons tous les talens [sic] que nous avons, les plaisirs que nous avons eus et mille autres, autres choses qui répandues dans notre vie nous ont donné l'existence la plus fortunée, et la plus enviable, que puissent avoir des jeunes personnes" ["Mama, I think that in losing our second mother, Mama Sophie, we have lost someone who loved us tenderly; and a dear benefactress who filled our lives with countless comforts from the time we were born, to whom we owe all the talents we possess, the pleasures we have known, and a thousand other things that, filling our lives, gave us the happiest and most enviable lives young people could ever have"].[7] One cannot imagine a greater tribute being paid to a mother and, though Cottin never brought children into the world, her devotion, sacrifice, and love for Julie's daughters earned her the right to the title of *maman* so generously bestowed here by a grateful adoptive child. Of all earthly honors, this was certainly Cottin's most prized.

The textual evidence I have examined in this study suggests that Sophie Cottin's struggle with her infertility closely matched the models provided by modern social psychology. A facile connection between the chronology of her textual production and the succeeding phases of the grieving cycle pointed out by Menning and others—surprise, denial, anger, isolation, guilt, and grief—would, of course, be misleading, but it is obvious that each of the elements in the cycle appears prominently at one point or another in her works. This was no doubt intensified by the acutely pronatalistic culture in which she lived and her own professed allegiance to the Rousseauian model of female domesticity. What is striking is the apparent developmental pattern of her oeuvre as a whole: one is left with the impression that writing functioned as autotherapy for her, allowing her to work through each phase until she reached a final resolution she could live with.

A brief examination of a significant recurring image in her texts, that of the tomb, helps elucidate this pattern. In each of her novels, Cottin includes a scene in which her main character either encounters or describes her encounter with a tomb. In every case, the tomb represents the past but, more importantly, it also symbolizes the Father: his presence, his power, and his law. In Cottin's first novel, her heroine Claire, in revolt against the Father, commits adultery on the very steps of his tomb as the culmination of her quest for personal plenitude. In striking contrast, her second heroine, Malvina, stands before her friend's tomb and swears allegiance to all it represents in terms of woman's maternal role. When Malvina becomes convinced that she has broken that vow, she kills herself. In the third novel, Amélie Mansfield, pregnant out of wedlock and angry at her victimization by a deceitful lover, swears to die on Father's tomb in symbolic rebellion against male perfidy and exploitation, which have robbed her of her own sense of identity. But in the fourth, an eternal virgin, inspired by the presence of a Christian warrior's tomb, successfully resists the passion of a forbidden lover and in so doing converts a non-Christian to the faith of her fathers. Cottin's last novel gives us a heroine who is a daughter first and foremost, a daughter dedicated to the redemption of the wronged Father. While on her way home with the document releasing her father from exile, which she has procured through enormous personal sacrifice, she stops to visit the tomb of another "father," this time a spiritual one, and pays homage to the old missionary who had extended his paternal protection over her as long as life would allow.

The evolution in this series of sepulchral encounters, spread over a ten-year writing career, appears to trace the various phases of Cottin's efforts to reconcile the realities of her "defectiveness" with the dominant cultural paradigm. The principal themes of the later texts and, we might add, her personal correspondence indicate that acceptance of her condition eventually replaced the anger and rebellion of the early years. But the texts remain as evidence of the difficulty of the struggle. If she could claim, as she did in the last year of her life, that she had finally anchored in calm waters, her novels attest to the violence of the storms endured along the way.

Notes

Introduction

1. Charles Augustin Sainte-Beuve, *Causeries du lundi*, vol. 11 (Paris: Garnier, n.d.), 488.
2. Leslie C. Sykes, *Madame Cottin* (Oxford: Basil, Blackwell, and Mott, 1949), 412–16. All subsequent references to this work will be cited parenthetically in the text using the abbreviated form *MC* followed by the page number.
3. Le Breton, describing Cottin's novels as a whole, wrote: "Elle a eu cet honneur et cette infortune que chacun de ses romans a été refait en tout ou en partie par quelque écrivain plus habile qu'elle et qui l'a fait oublier" ["She had the honor and the misfortune to have each of her novels redone completely or in part by some writer more talented than she and who caused her to be forgotten"] (*Le roman français au dix-neuvième siècle*, vol. 1, *Avant Balzac* [1901; reprint, Geneva: Slatkine, 1970], 93).
4. Sykes's work includes the most accurate biographical data currently available and extensive, though often edited, excerpts from her correspondence. This invaluable source has provided the factual information from which I have summarized Cottin's biography here, unless otherwise noted. Samia Spencer's summary of Cottin's life, which appears in *French Women Writers: A Bio-Bibliographical Source Book,* ed. Eva Martin Sartori and Dorothy Wynne Zimmerman (New York: Greenwood Press, 1991), 90–98, poses a problem in that Spencer neither quotes from Sykes's work nor includes his study in the bibliography accompanying the article and hence must be used with caution.
5. Scholarship on Cottin since the publication of Sykes's work has been spotty. Jean Gaulmier's two articles, "Sophie et ses malheurs; ou, Le romantisme du pathétique," *Romantisme* 3 (1970): 3–16, and "Roman et connotations sociales: *Mathilde* de Mme Cottin," in *Roman et société* (Paris: Colin, 1973), 7–17, helped to keep her name from disappearing altogether. Gaulmier was also responsible in large part for the only twentieth-century reprinting of a Cottin work, the 1976 Régine Deforges edition of *Claire d'Albe,* for which Gaulmier also wrote the introductory notes. Paul Pelckmans, in "L'impasse imaginaire: Notes sur la sensibilité familiale dans le roman français sous le Premier Empire," *Orbis Litterarum: International Review of Literary Studies* 34 (1979): 33–52, includes Cottin as part of his psychocritical study of the sentimental novel of the Napoleonic era. Janine Rossard devotes the first chapter of her book *Pudeur et romantisme* (Paris: Nizet, 1982) to an examination of the problem of chastity and female emancipation in *Claire d'Albe*. See also David J. Denby, "Le thème des croisades et l'héritage des lumières au début du 19e siècle," *Dix-huitième siècle* 19 (1987): 411–21; T. M. Pratt, "The Widow and the Crown: Madame Cottin and the Limits of Neoclassical Epic," *British Journal for Eighteenth-Century Studies* 9, no. 2 (1986): 197–203; and Colette Cazenobe, "Une

préromantique méconnue, Mme Cottin," *Travaux de littérature* 1 (1988): 175–202.

6. Frank Paul Bowman's summary of *Claire d'Albe* in *A New History of French Literature,* ed. Denis Hollier (Cambridge: Harvard University Press, 1989) and his recognition of Cottin's importance as a "portrayer of the plight of women" (602) are encouraging signs of a growing awareness of her work. Lynn Hunt in *The Family Romance of the French Revolution* (Berkeley: University of California Press, 1992) also uses *Claire d'Albe* as an example of postrevolutionary women's writing depicting the wife, who is "a tragic victim of the incompatibility between the demands of a conventional marriage and the impulses of a generous and true passion" (170). Here, as in the Bowman piece, the treatment of the novel and Cottin's work as a whole is very brief. Catherine Cusset's "Sophie Cottin; ou, L'écriture du déni," *Romantisme* 3, no. 77 (1992): 25–31, signals a renewed interest in Cottin's importance as a woman writing in "contradiction" with herself and her time, focusing on her struggle with the contradictions between sensuality and purity and between writing and mothering. Cusset spends little time, however, on *Claire d'Albe* and does not remark any significant difference between Cottin's first anonymously published novel and her subsequent novels, a difference that I attempt to demarcate in this study.

7. Judith Daniluk, Arthur Leader, and Patrick J. Taylor, "The Psychological Sequelae of Infertility," in *The Psychiatric Implications of Menstruation,* ed. Judith H. Gold (Washington, D.C.: American Psychiatric Press, 1985), 78.

8. Jane Read, *Counseling for Fertility Problems* (London: Sage, 1995), 39.

CHAPTER 1. EARLY LIFE OF SOPHIE COTTIN

1. For a general treatment of Rousseau's ideas on domesticity, see Barbara Corrado Pope, "The Influence of Rousseau's Ideology of Domesticity," in *Connecting Spheres: Women in the Western World, 1500 to Present,* ed. Marilyn J. Boxer and Jean H. Quataert (New York: Oxford University Press, 1987), 136–45.

2. Jean-Jacques Rousseau, *Emile; ou, De l'éducation* (Paris: Garnier, 1964), 455.

3. Ibid., 451.

4. Ibid., 477.

5. Jean Bethke Elshtain, *Public Man, Private Woman: Women in Social and Political Thought* (Princeton: Princeton University Press, 1981), 160–61.

6. Yvonne Knibiehler, "Les médecins et la 'nature féminine' au temps du Code civil," *Annales: Economies, sociétés, civilisations* 4 (July–August 1976): 824–45.

7. Ibid., 829.

8. Ibid., 830.

9. Quoted by Yvonne Knibiehler and Catherine Fouquet, *L'histoire des mères du moyen-âge à nos jours* (Paris: Montalba, 1980), 155.

10. Carol Duncan, "Happy Mothers and Other New Ideas in French Art," *Art Bulletin* 55, no. 4 (December 1973): 570.

11. Ibid., 577.

12. An excellent example is Elisabeth Vigée-Lebrun's official portrait of Marie Antoinette (1787) showing the queen surrounded by her three living children

and an empty cradle, signifying the death of an additional child. The portrait emphasizes the queen's maternal qualities.

13. Quoted by Duncan, "Happy Mothers," 570.
14. Ibid.
15. Quoted in ibid.
16. Interestingly, this description of Sophie bears a strong resemblance to the one given of her by Sainte-Beuve many years later. Sainte-Beuve, who was born in 1804 and hence would have never seen her, was forced to rely on secondhand information when he described her as follows: "Elle n'était pas belle, ni même agréable; blonde, un peu sur le roux, parlant peu, ayant l'air d'être toujours dans les espaces; mais elle avait de l'âme, du feu, de l'imagination" ["She was not pretty, not even attractive; blond, a little on the reddish side, speaking rarely, having the appearance of being always in the clouds; but she had spirit, fire, imagination"] (*Causeries*, 11:488).
17. The law authorizing the confiscation of property of those who had left France was passed on 9 February 1792.
18. Arnelle, *Une oubliée: Madame Cottin, d'après sa correspondance*, 2d ed. (Paris: Librairie Plon, 1914), 47–48. All subsequent references to this work will be cited parenthetically in the text using the abbreviated form *UO* followed by the page number.

Chapter 2. Infertility and Plenitude

1. For a general overview of the causes of amenorrhea, see Machelle M. Seibel, *Infertility: A Comprehensive Text* (Norwalk, Conn.: Appleton and Lange, 1990), 54–59. See also Michel Ferin, Raphael Jewelewicz, and Michelle Warren, *The Menstrual Cycle: Physiology, Reproductive Disorders, and Infertility* (New York: Oxford University Press, 1993), 129–30; and Rogerio A. Lobo et al., eds., *Mishell's Textbook of Infertility, Contraception, and Reproductive Endocrinology*, 4th ed. (Malden, Mass.: Blackwell, 1997), 301–10.

In individuals with normal breast and uterus development, blood tests are used to determine the source of the problem. If the prolactin level is abnormally high, then a pituitary tumor is suspected. If the prolactin level is normal, then the level of progesterone is evaluated. If the LH (luteinizing hormone) is high, then PCO is high or there is hypothalamic dysfunction. If FSH (follicle-stimulating hormone) is low, then the causes can be either a hypothalamic pituitary failure or ovarian failure (see Lobo et al., *Mishell's Textbook*, 309).

2. Henri de Latouche, ed., "Lettres inédites de Mme Cottin," *Revue de Paris* 18 (1830): 148–50.
3. Ibid., 148–49.
4. Jean-Louis Flandrin, *Families in Former Times: Kinship, Household, and Sexuality in Early Modern France*, trans. Richard Southern (Cambridge: Cambridge University Press, 1979), 179–80.
5. For this discussion I am indebted to Margaret Marsh and Wanda Ronner, *The Empty Cradle: Infertility in America from Colonial Times to the Present* (Baltimore: Johns Hopkins University Press, 1996), esp. 14, 15.
6. James Walker, *Inquiry into the Causes of Sterility in Both Sexes, with Its Method of Cure* (Philadelphia: E. Oswald, 1797), 7. All subsequent references to this work will be cited parenthetically in the text.
7. Marsh and Ronner, *Empty Cradle*, 17.

8. Ibid., 16.
9. Daniluk, Leader, and Taylor, "Psychological Sequelae of Infertility," 78–79.
10. Irina Pollard, *A Guide to Reproduction: Social Issues and Human Concerns* (Cambridge: Cambridge University Press, 1994), 6.
11. Barbara Menning, "The Emotional Needs of Infertile Couples," *Fertility and Sterility* 34 (October 1980): 313.
12. Ibid., 315.
13. Ibid., 316.
14. Read, *Counseling*, 26.
15. Ibid.
16. Menning, "Emotional Needs," 317.
17. Ibid.
18. In what he calls his "tasks of grieving," J. William Worden outlines the necessary steps in the grieving process and the consequences of failing to negotiate them:

> Task 1—Accepting the reality of the loss: denial must be overcome.
> Task 2—Working through the pain of the grief: if not worked through, it will manifest itself in some other way such as symptoms or behavior.
> Task 3—Adjusting to an environment in which the unborn child is missing: the loss of potential children is often accompanied by a loss of a sense of self and can have destructive effects on a couple's relationship.
> Task 4—Emotionally relocating the unborn child and moving on with life: patients must "learn to 're-invent' their lives without children, and to take pleasure and meaning from a world in which their own biological, and perhaps any, children are missing." (Read, *Counseling*, 30)

19. Sophie Cottin, *Oeuvres complètes*, 2 vols. (Paris: Ledentu, 1844), 1:398. All subsequent references to this work will be cited parenthetically in the text.
20. Madame de Genlis, "Madame Cotin [sic]," in *De l'influence des femmes sur la littérature française comme protectrices des lettres et comme auteurs; ou, Précis de l'histoire des femmes françaises les plus célèbres* (Paris: Maradan, 1811), 346. All subsequent references to this work will be cited parenthetically in the text.
21. Nancy Miller, *Subject to Change: Reading Feminist Writing* (New York: Columbia University Press, 1988), 127.

Chapter 3. Back in Step with Jean-Jacques: *Malvina*

1. Cottin later changed publishers, switching to Joseph Michaud to publish *Mathilde* (four thousand books in the first printing); she also sold Michaud the rights to *Claire d'Albe* since the Maradan edition had sold out. She agreed to revise *Malvina* and *Amélie Mansfield*, the rights to which Michaud had purchased from Maradan, in view of a second edition of both novels (Michaud and Cottin appear to have also paid off two notes Cottin held on Maradan for one thousand francs each). The total for this contract, concluded with Michaud in April 1805, was seven thousand francs. In 1806, Giguet and Michaud offered twelve hundred francs for the first edition of *Elisabeth*—which they found to be shorter than at first expected—and sixteen hundred francs for the rights to the book.

Chapter 4. The Anger of *Amélie Mansfield*

1. The wording in Cottin's letter suggests that André relayed the story of Charlotte Corday to her in his own words rather than an official or previously published version.
2. Menning, "Emotional Needs," 316.
3. Read, *Counseling*, 26.

Chapter 5. *Mathilde* and the Miracle of Bagnères

1. Latouche, "Lettres inédites," 149.
2. Ibid.
3. Ibid., 150.
4. Ibid.

Chapter 6. Filial Devotion in *Elisabeth*

1. The story appeared first in the *Journal des débats* and the *Publiciste* on 16 February 1805 and later in abridged form in the *Moniteur universel* and the *Bulletin de l'Europe* (see Sykes, *Madame Cottin*, 205–6).
2. "Pure et sans tache comme les anges, Elisabeth va participer à leur bonheur; elle va vivre comme eux d'innocence et d'amour. Ô amour! innocence! c'est assurément de votre éternelle union que se compose l'éternelle félicité" ["As pure and unspotted as the angels, Elisabeth will enjoy the happiness they know; she will live in love and innocence as they do. O love! innocence! eternally joined together, you surely define eternal happiness"] (1:539).
3. See Vladimir Propp, *Morphologie du conte* (Paris: Editions du Seuil, 1970).

Conclusion

1. Sainte-Beuve, *Causeries*, 11:488.
2. "Lettres et documents sur la maladie et la mort de Sophie Cottin," dossier cote 15985, Département des manuscrits (section occidentale), Bibliothèque Nationale, Paris.
3. Jean Caubet, *Sophie Cottin* (Tonneins: Jean Caubet, 1986), 40.
4. Sykes, *Madame Cottin*, 70.
5. Edward Shorter, *A History of Women's Bodies* (New York: Basic Books, 1982), 243–44.
6. Ibid., 243.
7. "Lettres et documents de Sophie Cottin," document 75, cote 15985.

Bibliography

Arnelle. *Une oubliée: Madame Cottin, d'après sa correspondance.* 2d ed. Paris: Librairie Plon, 1914.

Bowman, Frank Paul. "The Ideologists." In *A New History of French Literature,* edited by Denis Hollier, 596–602. Cambridge: Harvard University Press, 1989.

Caubet, Jean. *Sophie Cottin.* Tonneins: Jean Caubet, 1986.

Cazenobe, Colette. "Une préromantique méconnue, Mme Cottin." *Travaux de littérature* 1 (1988): 175–202.

Cottin, Sophie Risteau. *Correspondance.* Département des manuscrits (section occidentale), Bibliothèque Nationale, Paris.

———. *Oeuvres complètes.* 2 vols. Paris: Ledentu, 1844.

Cusset, Catherine. "Sophie Cottin; ou, L'écriture du déni." *Romantisme* 3, no. 77 (1992): 25–31.

Daniluk, Judith, Arthur Leader, and Patrick J. Taylor. "The Psychological Sequelae of Infertility." In *The Psychiatric Implications of Menstruation,* edited by Judith H. Gold, 75–85. Washington, D.C.: American Psychiatric Press, 1985.

Denby, David J. "Le thème des croisades et l'héritage des lumières au début du 19e siècle." *Dix-huitième siècle* 19 (1987): 411–21.

Duncan, Carol. "Happy Mothers and Other New Ideas in French Art." *Art Bulletin* 55 (December 1973): 570–83.

Elshtain, Jean Bethke. *Public Man, Private Woman: Women in Social and Political Thought.* Princeton: Princeton University Press, 1981.

Ferin, Michel, Raphael Jewelewicz, and Michelle Warren. *The Menstrual Cycle: Physiology, Reproductive Disorders, and Infertility.* New York: Oxford University Press, 1993.

Flandrin, Jean-Louis. *Families in Former Times: Kingship, Household, and Sexuality in Early Modern France.* Translated by Richard Southern. Cambridge: Cambridge University Press, 1979.

Frydman, René. *L'irrésistible désir de naissance.* Paris: Presses universitaires de France, 1986.

Gaulmier, Jean. "Roman et connotations sociales: *Mathilde* de Mme Cottin." In *Roman et société,* 7–17. Paris: Colin, 1973.

———. "Sophie et ses malheurs; ou, Le romantisme du pathétique." *Romantisme* 3 (1970): 3–16.

Genlis, Madame de. "Madame Cotin [sic]." In *De l'influence des femmes sur la littérature française comme protectrices des lettres et comme auteurs; ou, Précis de l'histoire des femmes françaises les plus célèbres.* Paris: Maradan, 1811.

Guerin, Guite. *L'enfant inconcevable: Histoires de femmes stériles*. Paris: Acropole, 1988.

Hunt, Lynn. *The Family Romance of the French Revolution*. Berkeley: University of California Press, 1992.

Knibiehler, Yvonne. "Les médecins et la 'nature féminine' au temps du Code civil." *Annales: Economies, sociétés, civilisations* 4 (July–August 1976): 824–45.

Knibiehler, Yvonne, and Catherine Fouquet. *L'histoire des mères du moyen-âge à nos jours*. Paris: Montalba, 1980.

Latouche, Henri de, ed. "Lettres inédites de Mme Cottin." *Revue de Paris* 18 (1830).

Le Breton, André. *Le roman français au dix-neuvième siècle. Vol. 1, Avant Balzac*. 1901. Reprint, Geneva: Slatkine, 1970.

Lobo, Rogerio A., et al., eds. *Mishell's Textbook of Infertility, Contraception, and Reproductive Endocrinology*. 4th ed. Malden, Mass.: Blackwell, 1997.

Marsh, Margaret, and Wanda Ronner. *The Empty Cradle: Infertility in America from Colonial Times to the Present*. Baltimore: Johns Hopkins University Press, 1996.

Menning, Barbara. "The Emotional Needs of Infertile Couples." *Fertility and Sterility* 34 (October 1980): 313–19.

Miller, Nancy. *Subject to Change: Reading Feminist Writing*. New York: Columbia University Press, 1988.

Monach, James H. *Childless, No Choice: The Experience of Involuntary Childlessness*. New York: Routledge, 1993.

Pelckmans, Paul. "L'impasse imaginaire: Notes sur la sensibilité familiale dans le roman français sous le Premier Empire." *Orbis Litterarum: International Review of Literary Studies* 34 (1979): 33–52.

Pollard, Irina. *A Guide to Reproduction: Social Issues and Human Concerns*. Cambridge: Cambridge University Press, 1994.

Pope, Barbara Corrado. "The Influence of Rousseau's Ideology of Domesticity." In *Connecting Spheres: Women in the Western World, 1500 to Present*, edited by Marilyn J. Boxer and Jean H. Quataert, 136–45. New York: Oxford University Press, 1987.

Pratt, T. M. "The Widow and the Crown: Madame Cottin and the Limits of Neoclassical Epic." *British Journal for Eighteenth-Century Studies* 9, no. 2 (1986): 197–203.

Read, Jane. *Counseling for Fertility Problems*. London: Sage, 1995.

Reboul, Jean. *Le désir, la mère, l'enfant*. Paris: Privat, 1986.

Rossard, Janine. *Pudeur et romantisme*. Paris: Nizet, 1982.

Rousseau, Jean-Jacques. *Emile; ou, De l'éducation*. Paris: Garnier, 1964.

Sainte-Beuve, Charles-Augustin. *Causeries du lundi*. 15 vols. Paris: Garnier, n.d.

Seibel, Machelle M. *Infertility: A Comprehensive Text*. Norwalk, Conn.: Appleton and Lange, 1990.

Shorter, Edward. *A History of Women's Bodies*. New York: Basic Books, 1982.

Spencer, Samia I. "Sophie Cottin." In *French Women Writers: A Bio-Bibliographical*

Source Book, edited by Eva Martin Sartori and Dorothy Wynne Zimmerman, 90–98. New York: Greenwood Press, 1991.

Sykes, Leslie C. *Madame Cottin*. Oxford: Basil, Blackwell, and Mott, 1949.

Walker, James. *Inquiry into the Causes of Sterility in Both Sexes, with Its Method of Cure*. Philadelphia: E. Oswald, 1797.

Index

Amenorrhea, 14, 50
Aristotle, 55
Arnelle, 116
Azaïs, Hyacinthe, 50, 107, 110, 113, 136, 137; *Essai sur le monde*, 136

Bagnères-de-Bigorre, France, 50; description of, 102, 105; *La Jouvence (the Fountain of Youth)* by Popineau in, *103*
Bordeaux, France, Risteau family connection with, 17, 24

Champlan, France: community of women in, 33; description of, 31
Chateaubriand, François-Auguste-René de, 31, 85–87, 110, 116
Corday, Charlotte, 82–83
Cottin, André (brother-in-law to SC), 80, 82, 83, 108, 115
Cottin, Jean-Paul-Marie (husband of SC): death of, 31; first impressions of Sophie Risteau, 24; marriage of, 27; political affiliations of, 29–30; political exile of, 30
Cottin, Sophie Risteau: on adoption of Julie Verdier's children, 34–35; *Amélie Mansfield*, summary and analysis of, 87–100; on *Atala*, 85–87; beginning of writing, 46; birth of, 17; childhood of, 17–18; *Claire d'Albe*, summary and analysis of, 62–70; death of, 155; death of husband, 31; death of mother, 33; on divorce, 38; education of, 23–24; *Elisabeth; ou, Les exilés de Sibérie*, summary and analysis of, 137–52; in exile during Revolution, 30, 71–72; on friendship with Julie Verdier, 33, 71; on her infertility, 51–53; liaison with Hyacinthe Azaïs, 110–14; *Malvina*, summary and analysis of, 75–81; on marriage, 25–26, 28–29, 47–48, 89; marriage of, 27–31; *Mathilde; ou, Mémoires tirés de l'histoire des croisades*, summary and analysis of, 116–33; monument to, *2*; move from Champlan, 43; on nature, 32; on notoriety, 136; on novels, 29; on pleasures of writing, 135; political status during Revolution, 32, 71–72; reaction to Jacques Lafargue's suicide, 41–43; reactions to Parisian life, 45–46; on religion, 104, 110–11, 136, 137; return to Champlan, 72 (1798), 112 (1804), 153 (1807); return of menstruation, 109–10; on Rousseau, 26–28; on suffering, 153–54; as surrogate mother, 35–37, 83–84, 104, 155–56; trip to Bagnères-de-Bigorre, 105; trip to Italy, 153–54; on women and politics, 40–41; on women and religion, 136–37; on women writers, 73–75, 136

Daniluk, Judith, 14, 59
Dentu, 115
Devaines, Jean, 84–85, 102
Diderot, Denis, 22
Duncan, Carol, 21–22

Elshtain, Jean, 20
Encyclopédie (1751–72), on woman's role, 21
Escoula, Jean, 2; monument to Sophie Cottin, *2*

Fragonard, Jean-Honoré, 22–23; *Heureuse Fécondité (Happy Fertility)*, 22–23, *23*

Genlis, Madame de, 68, 85, 87; on *Claire d'Albe*, 69–71; on *Elisabeth*, 137
Girardot, Antoine-Louis, 31, 32
Gramagnac, 33, 34, 37, 38–39

Greuze, Jean-Baptiste, 22; *Beloved Mother*, 22

Haller, Albrecht von, 57
Harvey, William, 55–56
Hippocrates, 21

Infertility: biblical stories of, 53–55; eighteenth-century science and, 55–59; psychological effects of, 14–15, 59–60; psychological stages of, 60–61; statistics on, 59

Jauge, Marguerite (sister-in-law of SC), 25, 72
Jauge, Théodore (brother-in-law of SC), 26

Knibiehler, Yvonne, 20–21

Lafargue, Agathe, 33
Lafargue, Félicité Vénès (cousin of SC), 33, 39, 41
Lafargue, Jacques, 36, 154; arrival at Champlan, 39; suicide of, 41
La Rochefoucauld, 20
Latouche, Henri de, 50
Leader, Arthur, 14, 59
Le Breton, André, 13
Lecourt, Anne (mother of SC), 17, 31
Ledentu, 116, 138
Leeuwenhoek, Anton van, 55, 57
Lemarcis, Constant, 47, 62
Lemarcis, Mélanie, 109, 153

Maradan, 62, 80, 81, 100
Marat, Jean-Paul, 82
Marsh, Margaret, 58
Marten, John, 56
Menning, Barbara, 59–60
Meung, Jean de, 20
Michaud, Joseph, 18, 114–15, 134
Miller, Nancy, 70
Molière, 20
Montaigne, Michel de, 20

Pastoret, Madame de, 108, 112
Pelet, Amable, 43, 44–45
Popineau, 103; *La Jouvence (the Fountain of Youth)*, 103

Read, Jane, 15, 61
Risteau, Jacques (father of SC), 17, 30
Ronner, Wanda, 58
Rousseau, Jean-Jacques: *Confessions*, 27; *Emile*, 18–19, 20, 28; *La nouvelle Héloïse*, 27, 28, 65–66; pronatalism and, 14; "separate spheres" doctrine of, 23; on woman's role in society, 18–20
Roussel, Pierre: predestination of woman to maternity, 20–21; *Système physique et moral de la femme* (1775), 20

Sainte-Beuve, Charles Augustin, 13, 154
Salut hot springs (Thermes du Salut), 105, *107*
Shorter, Edward, 155
Soubies, Fanny, 105
Soubies, François-Marie, 105
Spallanzani, Lazzaro, 57
Staël, Madame de, 26; *Lettres sur le caractère et les ouvrages de J.-J. Rousseau*, 26–27
Sykes, Leslie C., 13, 15–16, 18, 47, 50, 61, 83, 155; on Cottin's cause of death, 155; *Madame Cottin*, 13, 15–16

Taylor, Patrick J., 14, 59
Thermes du Salut, 105, *107*
Tonneins, 17, 38, 102, 104, 135

Vallon du Salut, *106*
Verdier, Delphine (daughter of Julie Verdier), 28, 33, 104, 105, 107, 155
Verdier, Elisa (daughter of Julie Verdier), 33, 104, 105
Verdier, Julie Vénès (cousin of SC), 14, 17, 25, 27, 31, 33; health problems of, 72, 83, 104, 108, 109
Verdier, Mathilde (daughter of Julie Verdier), 35, 104, 108
Verdier, Pierre, 34, 37, 38, 102, 135
Virey, Julien Joseph: definition of woman's role, 21; *Dictionnaire des sciences médicales* (1812–22), 21

Walker, James, 56; *Inquiry into the Causes of Sterility in Both Sexes* (1797), 56–59

OHIO UNIVERSITY LIBRARY
Please return this book as soon as you have finished with it. In order to avoid a fine it must date stamp